Heal Your Neck Issues

and Let Your

Throat

Chakra

Shine

The Spiritual Guide to
Moving Forward Pain-Free

CHERYL STELTE

ISBN: 978-19-5-315321-0

Published by

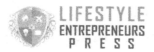

If you are interested in publishing through Lifestyle Entrepreneurs Press,
write to: *Publishing@LifestyleEntrepreneursPress.com*

Publications or foreign rights acquisition of our catalog books.
Learn More: *www.LifestyleEntrepreneursPress.com*

Printed in the USA

Advance Praise

"HEAL YOUR NECK ISSUES and Let Your THROAT CHAKRA SHINE Neck issues are more than common in today's world. They are familiar to men and women, children and babies, and also the geriatric population. There are many different ways these neck issues can be treated.

Cheryl Stelte points in the title of her book which way her treatment is directed: how to heal neck pain by using spiritual energy to connect the mind and heart through the bottleneck of the throat. Cheryl Stelte will not be treating our neck issues with medications, chiropractic adjustments or fascia alignments. By mentioning the word "chakra," she directs us toward meditation and ancient wisdom.

The throat chakra represents a portal for deep and direct connection to the spiritual world. It is by having knowledge about the throat chakra, and skill in using that knowledge, that the healing process can be managed. The throat chakra is the transition region where some of the cranial nerves enter the spine, and through which the vagus nerve connects to the larynx, inner ears, the eyes, and all the organs in the body including the lungs, the heart, stomach, intestines, bladder and sexual organs. As this book explains, this is a key area for physical, emotional and spiritual health.

Cheryl's incredible, heart-breaking stories will keep you spellbound reading this book. A near-death experience in Africa and the suicide of her brother propelled her on a decade-long search to heal. Her exotic life experiences gave her insight on how her neck issues were really connected with the throat chakra, and this is an insight for us all.

The healing tools Cheryl found for the deep injuries of her throat center are put together in this book as a rare combination which is unique to Cheryl Stelte's work. Cheryl is a master of Shamanism (as taught at the Foundation for Shamanic Studies) who knows how to work with power animals for deep inner transformation. Cheryl is also, and chiefly, a master of Heart Rhythm Meditation as taught at the iam-Heart school. Cheryl knows the techniques that enable her to deeply connect with her clients. As she explains, she experiences within herself the pain of the client and the cause of that pain, and has the knowledge to find very personal ways for healing the throat chakras of her clients. Cheryl's manner is insightful, confident and forthcoming.

Through her very personal style it will be easy to find trust in your relationship with Cheryl and to find your next step (and hopefully your last step) in healing your neck and throat issues."

—Susanna & Puran Bair
Co-Authors of *Living From The Heart, Energize Your Heart, and Follow Your Heart*

I have found Cheryl Stelte's "Heal Your Neck Pain and Let Your Throat Chakra Shine" book and program extremely helpful for me on multiple levels including; the physical, emotional, practical and spiritual. Prior to working with Cheryl, I was experiencing problems on each of these levels.

Physically, I had suffered from a chronically stiff neck which was often painful. I also experienced chronic back pain. I had gone to my chiropractor once a month for years. These visits provided temporary relief, but if I skipped a few visits then the pain always returned. The pain was getting worse as I aged so I began attributing my aches and pains as an inevitable by-product of getting older. After working with Cheryl in her program my chronic pain disappeared. Although, I still occasionally experience a flare up, I can easily cure the aches by doing the practices that I learned from her. It is a great relief to be pain free. I had gotten so used to living with the pain that I didn't realize what a tremendous burden I had until it was lifted.

Through an intense process of wound healing using many of the methods described in her book I was able to heal the emotional wounds that were causing me such difficulties in a few long term relationships. I was able to stop the pattern of repetitive unconscious behaviors that were holding me back and causing both me and those around me such distress. I am a much happier person now. I find that my happiness is reflected back to me more and more by the people that I work and recreate with.

On the practical, meaning career, Cheryl's training and support helped to give me the strength, courage and insight that I needed to clean house in my business and to embark on a program of rebirth and re-creation of my business and career. Now I am unifying my economic life more closely with my life's purpose.

Spiritually, I discovered that my wounds were holding me back from accepting my own power, guidance and purpose. I am now able to take full responsibility for my own spiritual progress. I will also be able to become a great teacher and healer - one who channels my inner being and deep purpose.

I am very grateful for Cheryl's pushing the boundaries of self-healing and improvement in such a dramatic and beneficial manner. I highly recommend her book and her program to you.

—John Happel
Business owner and meditation teacher

"In the midst of great change in my life I was fortunate to embark on healing work with Cheryl. Embodying the energies of healer / best friend / mother / cheerleader, her rich and varied training – synthesized into a deep internal knowing – gained my trust immediately. Intensely present, nothing wild that comes up fazes her, and she shares in my gains with gusto. I have <u>never</u> had such relief from physical pain and mental torment after decades of working with chiropractic, yoga, acupuncture, nutrition, even meditation. In class or in individual sessions, her sensitivity and skill, matched by her unwavering support, has allowed me to grow beyond what I thought possible, and in an exceptionally short time. One of my most significant "ah-ha" moments ever came to consciousness through participating in her intensely gratifying 5th Chakra class. And I have lifelong tools to use on my own now that we got through the darkest, hardest, scariest part of the journey together. Imagine knowing you can help yourself move beyond chronic pain and self-soothe in the most troubling situations, when previously you thought there was no way. It is the hardest work I've ever done, but my resilience, outlook in the present and for the future, relief from pain and renewed physical strength, self-respect and assuredness are beyond measure. And this, all while a viral pandemic swept through the world."

—Wendy Weiss,
Commercial Realtor

"Cheryl's book and companion program was the most impactful forward moving course I've ever taken. The amount of growth and healing that naturally occurred without effort was mind-boggling. Not only did I have huge throat chakra healing and awareness, my first three chakras had major healing too. It's hard to understand how meeting with Cheryl and doing her meditations can have such an impact resulting in massive change for the better. I am so THRILLED by the course and my outcome, I'm taking the 9 month throat chakra course with Cheryl too. The best course I've ever taken for healing. Cheryl is one of the most generous teachers I've ever had the pleasure of witnessing. I highly recommend this book and program for anyone who is looking for positive change, rapidly without pain and agony!"

—Diane Boerner
Registered Nurse of 41 years!

"Through Cheryl's book and under her caring guidance, I have brought love, healing, forgiveness, and compassion to myself and my beautiful inner child. The guided meditations, while intense, were so incredibly helpful in releasing a lot of what is stopping me from living my life out loud and on my terms. It's a daily practice doing these meditations but the breakthroughs and freedom you get after deeply clearing long held wounds is worth it. While working through this program, I have taken steps to put my creative writing out into the world and restored hope to my heart. Thanks to Cheryl, I am on the right path where I can proudly shine my inner starlight, speak my truth, and express myself with nothing and no one holding me back."

—Aleka Allen

"I just completed Cheryl's book and 8 week ccourse. Most of my life, and especially for the last year, I have had severe neck issues. After after doing the directed meditations and the class work and the stretches, along with the wonderful personal healing sessions, I am happy to say that my neck pain is almost completely gone!.

Through Cheryl's intuitive guidance and accurate expla-nainations I have been able to see into myself deeper than ever before and have developed a whole new relationship with my Chakras. After 15 years of intense inner work I have reached a new level of self communication and a clearer connection to my cosmic roots.

Thank you, Cheryl. From the bottom of my Heart."

—John Comunale,
Artist and Owner of Sculptural Concepts

Author Cheryl Stelte's "Heal Your Neck Issues and Let Your Throat Chakra Shine" caught my attention. I have heard great reviews of author Cheryl Stelte and her many, many successful achievements. I knew nothing about Chakras, and thought this would be an interesting book to read. Cheryl shares her inner most ups and downs of her past 25 years of life traveling to many parts of the world to gain knowledge and wisdom for her own life, and to share with others.

Much to my delight, from the very beginning of this book Cheryle caught my inner most interest. I felt I was on each of her journeys traveling the world learning many different healing avenues which she lovingly captured and is sharing in this book.

Throughout this book I felt a strong connection with Cheryl and realized I did have Chakra and wanted her to guide me through the learning cycle. Cheryl's writing is soft, calming and clearly written with compassion and love, she shares honestly and openly.

As my reading continued, I realized Cheryl was with me spiritually, it was almost impossible to put this book down and tend to my daily chores. I quickly realized I want Cheryl to guide me in Meditation and Chakra healing.

I urge you to read Cheryl's book, if not for Meditation or Chakra healing, simply to enjoy this remarkable woman's journey through her past 25 years which is truly inspirational. It will leave you a different person.

—Sheila B
—Kelowna BC, Canada

I dedicate this book to Dan, Charla, and Amin
for all the love that we share.

Contents

Chapter 1

Why It's so Important to Heal Your Neck Issues

"Healing may not be so much about getting better, as about letting go of everything that isn't you – all of the expectations, all of the beliefs – and becoming who you are."

—Rachel Naomi Remen

It was early one morning when the pain started. I was getting ready for work and sat on the edge of my bed when I started to feel pain developing in my neck. I thought, "Oh no, here we go again with another kink in my neck." The pain rapidly increased in intensity and fear began to overwhelm me. That pain had never happened before. The pain grew and grew until it was excruciating. Any movement made it worse. I had no idea how to relieve the pain and considered going to the doctor or the emergency room. I wondered what doctors would do and knew I would likely be given medication.

I had never been to a chiropractor and somehow knew it was time to go. I called and left a message at the nearest chiropractic office and was grateful they returned my call right after they opened. The chiropractor even got me in that morning. I phoned in sick to work and had to cancel all my appointments. I could barely move, and driving was next to impossible. Before leaving my house, I applied ice, but it did not help at all.

The diagnosis was a pinched nerve in my neck. I spent five days and nights in bed and visited the chiropractor every few days during and following that time. I never would have guessed that it would take years to fully recover. I had no idea what caused the pain and certainly did not expect it to have anything to do with my emotions or spirituality. I didn't know then that neck pain is related to the throat chakra. My severe neck pain was a way of my body telling me that I had serious throat chakra issues.

Obviously, you picked up this book because you are experiencing some sort of neck pain, tension, soreness, or some sort of neck issues, but why *this* book? If you ended up like me, trying various alternative or healing therapies, with or without western medicine, and still were never able to eliminate your neck pain, you started to look further. You learned that energy, chakras, and spirituality are becoming more and more attractive as a path worth pursuing for many reasons. You have at least begun to see that maybe your constant or recurring neck pain has more to do with what has happened or what is happening in your subconscious and/or your emotions than what is happening physically. The real root cause of your neck pain is illusory, and the more you learn about the chakras and specifically the throat chakra, you became quite aware that there are some related areas that are in need of healing. Maybe you already experienced some healing and want to go deeper, see what else is out there, and create more healing.

At the same time that you are experiencing an ongoing or occasional sore neck or various neck issues, you feel stuck in your life, career, relationship, and health. You want to move forward, and while you try different approaches, you just don't get that far. Maybe you're just not that clear on where you want to get to. How can you possibly move forward if you don't know where forward is? You know there is more to life than the life you are living, and you just need a framework to get you there.

After many years of working on my throat chakra, I continued to train in meditation, reiki, acupressure, various energy healing, and shamanism, and finally got to the bottom of all my neck issues and pain. I decided to make a career out of helping others heal their throat chakra and move forward in life. One of my clients went to the chiropractor for over thirty years for his neck and back pain, so I suggested a number of the practices in this book and did some energetic healing sessions on him. Within a few months, he stopped going to the chiropractor, and his pain was gone. My client thought he would be going to the chiropractor for the rest of his life and that his pain had become age-related. He was sixty-four years old and has never looked back. Now, if he feels any pain in his neck or back, he does the practices to move beyond the emotional or spiritual cause, and when he needs help, he occasionally requests an energetic healing from me.

This book is written to help you understand yourself more fully as not only a physical being but also as an energetic, emotional, and spiritual being. The teachings here contain a toolkit of practices to help you get to the root cause of your neck pain and all that keeps you stuck in your life. This is a fairly intense path for those who are willing to, as Susan Jeffers says, "feel the fear and do it anyway."

Susan Jeffers was an American psychologist and author, and her book *Feel the Fear and Do It Anyway* helped me enhance my daily meditating practice and become more of my true self. That was back in 1998, and I can't say how grateful I am and how many times I have recommended her book. What I discovered since then is that affirmations work very well in helping to change our thoughts, and it is a lot of work. I have also found that working in the heart and the energy centers, we are able to access the root or cause of our detrimental thoughts and move through our emotions and spiritual blocks which then create significant and permanent change in our thoughts and behaviors without the daily reminders to think differently.

The chapters in this book provide a step-by-step process for you to uncover what is hidden in your subconscious that contributes to the pain and problems you experience today. Once uncovered, you will learn to accept and heal the past, change limiting beliefs and values, heal core wounds, and move beyond the obstacles that cause pain and get in your way. This process will then assist you in a wonderful process of self-discovery and help you become more of who you truly are, guiding and supporting you in taking steps forward in your life that feel impossible right now.

This book is designed to help you change your life permanently and guide you through the process of becoming pain-free. You know there is more to your neck pain than you currently realize, and you know there is a much greater life for you out there than the one you live now. This process creates changes within you at different levels, and doors to new opportunities and possibilities that don't currently exist will open. Life will become more meaningful in areas of work, relationships, health, and spirituality.

My experience is that the longer we continue to try to live with the pain and stay stuck in our lives, the harder it is to create lasting change for the better. It's pretty hard to live our lives fully and joyfully in the ways we were meant to with constant or recurring neck pain. Our own sense of well-being takes a hit every time we wake up with pain or reinjure ourselves. Living in pain and feeling stuck in life lowers confidence and leads to lack of motivation, depression, inability to participate fully in life, as well as feelings of hopelessness, helplessness, unworthiness, and despair. We don't know how to, or can't seem to, pursue our dreams, create the relationships we desire, or even imagine living life fully with contentment or happiness, and we fear that it will be like this forever ensues.

I believe that there are people out there who need you and all that you came here to do. Whether you are an artist, writer, teacher, technician, engineer, scientist, surfer, or politician, a part of humanity needs you in a unique way, in the particular expression of the one and only you. Your unique soul was born into your unique body so that you can live on this earth plane, expressing who you truly are in your own unique way. When the student is ready, the teacher appears. Let this book serve you the way you would love it to serve you. I will do my best as your guide, your mentor or coach, and the person who's got your back (and your neck) and absolutely your best interest at heart.

Heal your neck pain and let your throat chakra shine!

Chapter 2:

How Life's Struggles Brought Me to Purpose

"The purpose of our lives is to give birth to the best which is within us"
—Marianne Williamson

I first began meditating twenty-five years ago to end depression and get off antidepressants, and it worked so well, I got off the antidepressants in a matter of months and have never looked back. I knew I had to keep meditating to keep depression away, and it wasn't until later that I realized meditation could help me in many other ways, including healing my neck pain and throat chakra issues.

When I first had my neck injury, I didn't think for a moment that my meditation practice could help heal my neck. Once I started to read books on the chakras and working with these amazing energy centers, I had many great and encouraging experiences, but there was nothing that I read or learned that led me to believe that meditating on the chakras could heal pain. I did notice that my chronic tinnitus and laryngitis stopped along with the depression. My neck pain did decrease, but I did not make the connection, and I thought it was simply the yoga that was helping my neck pain. As I had a number of throat chakra issues, I noticed that the more I meditated on my throat chakra, the more I was able to speak my truth and the more confident, expressive, clear I became about the direction I wanted my life to take. My life continued to improve and the more it improved, the less neck pain I experienced. It wasn't until a few years later when I was meditating and I experienced a snake around my neck that I began to see the connection, but I'm getting ahead of myself. More on that later!

There are so many symptoms of throat chakra issues that I think I could almost write an entire book on them. The throat chakra includes the ears, jaw, mouth, neck, top of the shoulders, thyroid, throat, atlas, and more. Many people experience neck pain or tension, thyroid issues, hearing loss, and problems with teeth or jaw and shoulder pain when they have throat chakra issues. To me, it is the most difficult chakra to heal and develop, but working to heal and empower it is so worthwhile, and I feel such a strong calling to help others do the same. My wish is to save you a great deal of time in healing and developing your throat chakra and share with you the most powerful practices of healing and empowerment. You deserve it; you have something great to share with the world, and it's your throat chakra that naturally wants to express it. Through this process, I learned so much about my humanity and the great importance of the throat chakra.

If you feel ready, I would love to help you navigate your own healing of this vital center so that you may move forward, creating a pain-free existence, more meaningful work and relationships, and an expression of your truth and ultimately your soul's purpose.

My Story

When my kids were twelve and fourteen, I took them to San Diego for summer vacation. We went with my dad, his wife, and her two kids. I saw people having a great time boogie boarding and just had to get in on the action. I bought one for myself and each of my kids, and off we went. I didn't read the sign about riptides, as it was small and off to the side. We headed out to the water and had a fantastic time when suddenly a big wave caught me, and I smashed to the bottom of the ocean, hitting my head and hurting my neck. It didn't hurt for too long, and I continued to boogie board. We started to realize, when the lifeguard blew his whistle, everyone had stopped boogie boarding because of the riptides. My family and I had to ask someone on the beach what a riptide was to figure this out – *duh.* But by that time, I had injured my neck a number of times. The pain grew to the point of ending up with a pinched nerve in my neck. It was excruciating for about a week, even with the help of a chiropractic. As time went on, I experienced more neck pain, showing my poor discernment of a common throat chakra issue.

Over the years, I experienced a great deal of self-doubt, thinking that others were better than me and that I wasn't good or worth enough. I often followed other's advice before my own and entered into relationships that were not good for me, even though my initial hunch was to not even entertain the idea. I couldn't trust my own truth, my own intuition, as well as I would have liked to, which made discernment challenging. These feelings were rooted in early childhood as I felt like I never really fit in. I often found myself feeling unfulfilled and stuck, and as a result, I suffered through years of infrequent and then chronic neck pain.

My road to recovery was long and grueling. At that time in my life, I also experienced serious hearing loss and teeth problems. Whenever I saw myself in the reflection of a building or a mirror in a public place, I noticed that my shoulders were always drooping forward. And after I divorced my ex-husband, I could not find a man with whom I could have a healthy relationship. However, over the years, I steadily began to choose men that were healthier emotionally and mentally, and now I am married to such a wonderful and amazing man – my best friend ever. My neck pain completely disappeared, and while my hearing didn't return permanently, it stopped declining and hasn't changed at all in over ten years.

We often develop patterns in our behavior that stem from early emotional wounds created within the families we grew up with. It is often the people who love us the most that make these marks on us. These marks remain in the subconscious until we choose to see these hurts and heal them. Our soul chooses our parents; our parents don't choose us. We all know what we are in for before we are born; your soul accepts the human challenges that help you grow to express your soul's purpose one day.

Everything that has gotten in my way and all the difficulties I experienced in my family of origin served me. Were my parents bad people? Absolutely not. Did I go through a period of feeling like they were bad people? Yes, somewhat (I'm sorry, Mom and Dad; I love you so much). I went through a period where I looked at all the wounds of my early childhood and sat in the victim role for a while. I needed to feel the pain so that I could heal it and overcome it. I had to heal this pain to move into forgiveness, and then later, I became grateful for all the good and bad in my childhood, as it made me become who I am today.

The Universe knows your purpose, and life would not be what it is without challenges. We have to experience the low times to fully enjoy the high times. It is through feeling our pain fully that we are able to forgive. My experience is that the long way to do this is through talking about it (or talk therapy), and the expedited way is through powerful meditation techniques and energy healing. The type of meditation I use in this book helps heal so quickly because we get to the energetic wound and can transform it quickly, resulting in great healing. The heart is more than just a physical organ pumping blood; it is an emotional and energetic center that is designed to feel. That's why we have a heart.

Most societies do not support feeling emotions fully, let alone expressing them fully, so we learn to stuff emotions down and deny and ignore them. About ten years ago when my neck pain was getting to be much better, I was doing some serious inner child work and remember going through my childhood birthday cards that my beloved mother saved for me and pulled them out of the beautiful box where my mother so lovingly placed special mementos from my childhood. I read the cards from birth to around age eight. From birth to age seven, not one family member signed their name with the word "love" – not one – not my grandparents, aunts, or uncles. I was so dismayed.

At the time, it felt as if I had missed out on the love I needed. I cried my tears and felt a little better. It wasn't until I breathed these feelings of regret and loss into my meditations that I moved from feeling sorry for myself to understanding that it was just a sign of the times – a sign of the stage of human evolution in that era. In my heart, I could feel how much my family loved me, but their capacity to express it was limited through throat chakra issues. Thank goodness my family and much of humanity have evolved to express love more freely and unconditionally.

My parents, who absolutely did their very best and were amazing and wonderful parents in many ways, were fairly controlling. At a young age I married a controlling man. In turn, we were both controlling parents, and I still apologize about this to my adult kids today. My children are just so loving, compassionate, and forgiving. I am so encouraged by young people today and how loving they are with their children.

Being around controlling people stifles the throat chakra. We are afraid to express what's in our hearts and express our truths. At the same time, people who are controlling have throat chakra issues. The need for control is often rooted in fear – fear of not being heard or seen or even understood. For years, I worked on trying to discover what was in my heart and what was true for me. Taking this knowledge and learning to express it without fear were big hurdles.

I used to have trouble speaking in large groups. There was a time when I worked for a renovation company and my boss Larry wanted me to do a radio show with him as a way of increasing business. It felt like he wanted to make me famous, and I wanted no part of it. Throat chakra issues can be expressed by someone talking way too much, all the time, because they didn't feel seen or heard well in childhood, and that was definitely me as a kid and young adult. The same issue of not feeling seen or heard can be expressed by someone who hardly speaks at all. They may have given up on being seen or heard. Of course, this does not mean that this applies to everyone. One must explore one's own throat chakra.

My biggest fear, that has taken me the longest to get over, is fear of success or fear of expressing my greatness. If you knew me then, you likely would not have seen it. I appeared fairly confident to the outside world. I became one of a small group of experts in solving moisture problems in people's homes. I lived in Victoria, Canada, where moisture problems were common and often affected children's respiratory health. I was passionate about turning sick homes into healthy homes, and Larry wanted to capitalize on that. With my throat chakra issues, I didn't want to be seen or recognized even though I eventually went along with him and did the radio show for over a year. It was like I wanted to get the message of my heart out but not be recognized for it.

There are always some things that are not worth saying, and I do my best to say what I need to say with compassion, understanding, and respect for others. I learned to practice discernment, when to listen, and when to speak. Now, I have no problem expressing what is in my heart and what is true for me, and my hope is that expressing myself encourages others to do the same.

I started reading many self-help books as I believed I could create the change I desired. After working with Susan Jeffers' book, I bought a book on the chakras and worked with that for some time. I purchased more books on the chakras and studied, learned, and meditated. I was mostly focused on the lower chakras because the issues I had in my lower chakras felt like the most important to heal at that time but for some reason didn't acquire the skills to really heal my throat chakra. My work on the lower chakras supported my work on the throat chakra later. I knew when it was time to focus there.

I was meditating one day when I felt pressure and tightening around my neck. This was new, and as the sensations increased and became more uncomfortable, I had a visual of a blue snake wrapped tightly around my neck. What a metaphor it was for me. At first, I was startled and tried to energetically remove it. My efforts were ineffective, and then I realized the snake was there to get my attention and to help me work with my throat chakra. I worked with that snake, energetically, at length, healing what was ready to be healed, integrating for long periods of time, and then moving to the next level. This on and off process took years, and I have developed and learned methods to move through this so much faster and efficiently.

I had tinnitus, or loud ringing in the ears, as a child. It was often so loud it was painful. By the time I was in my thirties, I experienced various sounds of tinnitus. I would hear ringing, buzzing, clicking, and hissing. The ringing was always the most uncomfortable, but the clicking continued to happen primarily when I was meditating. I would want to stop meditating because it was such a distraction, but I knew I had to persevere. I started to breathe into the sound and over months, it slowly disappeared altogether. Through meditation, all tinnitus symptoms completely vanished, and I haven't suffered from tinnitus for over twenty years.

I had hearing loss since I was in my early twenties, and it became pretty serious by the time I was in my mid-thirties; in fact, I went through a period of about three months where my hearing came back one hundred percent. It was a miraculous time, but I wasn't able to maintain it long-term.

I learned about and practiced Peter Levine's somatic experiencing with a practitioner and on my own in my meditations. Peter Levine is an author and the founder of The Somatic Experiencing Trauma Institute, which continues his ground-breaking research into the effects of trauma and stress on the body and the nervous system. One day while practicing this method on myself (which is not what it was intended for), I had one of the most intense meditations of my life. I felt like a huge electric cable went through my body vertically, and I shook, vibrated, and convulsed for about an hour and a half. I know this is certainly not the intention of Peter Levine's work, and as I was doing this alone, I was not practicing with a skilled practitioner on that day. After that, I was so wiped out that I slept for about three hours. By dinner time, I realized my hearing returned, and I heard sounds so sharply – sounds that I hadn't heard in years. I could hear my hair rubbing on my jacket and my footsteps on the pavement.

The following day, I went for a walk at East Sooke Park which is on Vancouver Island where I loved living for twenty-four years. The parking lot is quite a distance from the ocean, and I remember hearing the ocean long before I would have in the past. It was such an exciting time for me, and I thought I would be like that forever. Instead of constantly saying, "Pardon me?" to people, I asked them to whisper to me because, for the first time in years, I could hear whispers. My improved hearing lasted about three months, and I realize now that I didn't have the capacity to maintain it. My remaining unhealed throat chakra issues continued to creep back, and my hearing deteriorated again. I had hoped that I would return to this heightened state of hearing permanently but have not been able to hold that. Specialists could not understand or explain what happened, but I have not lost hope. The good news is that while my hearing continued to deteriorate for fifteen years, after that time, my hearing stopped deteriorating and has not worsened at all in the last twenty years, which is unusual for hearing loss.

I was later guided to go back to school to study interior design. I clearly remember going to the drugstore to pick up a few things, and on my way out the door, there was an adult education booklet sitting in a stand that grabbed my attention. I looked over at it and thought, "I'm not taking any classes; I'm not going back to school."

I was a single mother doing it all on my own and was doing okay financially. I remember being so happy when I started to make enough money to be able to take my kids out to restaurants and buy them some brand name clothes. At one time, the money I made was just enough to get food on the table. I had no intention of going back to school, but I walked through the automatic door just to be pulled right back into the store. I stood in front of the stack of course calendars and just stared at them. I kept repeating to myself, "I'm not going back to school. This is stupid; I'm not going to school."

However, the calendar just kept calling my name, so I finally surrendered and said, "Fine!" I picked the calendar up and put it in my bag. Once home, I went to my meditation room – yes, I was blessed with a meditation room off my bedroom where I meditated daily and led meditations for friends. I made myself a cup of tea and took the course calendar in there with me. I opened it up to a random page, and there it was, a program called "the Business of Interior Design."

I repeated, "I am not going back to school." I grew up with my parents continuously re-decorating the house and my ex-husband and I enjoyed decorating our homes. As a single mother, I painted walls and doors and sewed custom drapes and blinds, throw pillows, shower curtains, bedding, and even slipcovers. I learned how to install wood trim, replacing all the baseboards and door and window casings in two houses. At age thirteen, my son and I replaced all the linoleum in our duplex with wood flooring. It was a lifelong hobby, not a career. The long and the short of it was that after attending an info session and going to the bank to borrow money, I was enrolled in the program and graduated at the top of the class. I had to laugh because the bank even loaned me the money to make the loan payments while I was in school with absolutely no collateral security.

Once I graduated, I went for one interview with a fairly prestigious design firm and the owner, who interviewed me, was over half an hour late. I left right when she arrived, knowing it wasn't meant to be. I toyed with the idea of starting my own business. I was new to interior design and had little business experience, but I did it anyway. I maxed out my credit cards and got new cards and gave myself one year to make a go of it. I told my kids money was going to continue to be tight for a while. I worked my butt off, and just when I felt like giving up, around the nine- or tenth-month mark, I got a big job that covered more than one month's living expenses. With this job, I was able to continue to pay all the bills going forward.

Looking back, I realize all my throat chakra issues in that business. I didn't advertise and built my business by word-of-mouth. I see how I didn't charge enough for my services for years and realize now it was because of my hidden low self-worth. I wasn't able to receive compliments. I even remember one of my clients often offering her help in taking my samples back out to my vehicle. I never accepted this kind offer, and one day, she said to me, "Cheryl, it's nice for the other person to have their offer of help accepted. It gives them a good feeling."

I could easily offer my help for others but not receive help. For a long time, I remembered that and tried to receive help, but it usually felt uncomfortable. This attitude reflected my wounds, and I am grateful that meditation has helped me so much that now I am able to receive and give equally.

I was on a strong spiritual path through this time, studying with Denise Linn, author and world-acclaimed expert in Feng Shui and space clearing, and incorporating her work of interior alignment into my business. My tag line for Stelte

Design was *"Designing for the Soul,"* so Denise's Feng Shui training fit that to a certain extent. I brought in a lot of meditation where I received guidance for my clients and some shamanism as well. Doing this work for my clients helped to heal my neck pain and throat chakra issues because I was expressing part of my soul's purpose. I didn't realize it at the time, but it is more than clear now. Every year I let my throat chakra shine in this way, my neck pain diminished. I started my business twenty years ago, and I see now how I was a bit ahead of the times. I had a small percentage of clients who wanted to work at a spiritual level, but I was in heaven when I worked with the ones who did, and we always achieved great success.

I had friends and clients who suggested I teach, and I never thought I had what it took. My best friend often told me, "You are a spiritual teacher and a healer. Look at all you do: you meditate, you are a shaman, and you bring your spirituality into everything you do." I would always respond by saying, "I have enough trouble healing myself, let alone trying to help others do the same." Looking back, that comment seems humorous because now it's all I want to do, and making the choice to become the spiritual teacher, healer, and coach that I am was one of the best things I have ever done.

I never experience neck pain and haven't for years. If I ever even feel a tinge of anything, I address it right away so I don't need to suffer. I can't say enough about how much I value working on the throat chakra. I do my stretches a few times a week and meditate on all my chakras daily, occasionally incorporating Heart-Centered Shamanism as well as do things that express who I truly am and my soul's purpose. It

19

has not been easy, but it has been so worthwhile. It is one thing to heal your wounds and it is something else to take action steps and speak your truth.

Just before I started writing this chapter, my screen saver changed to a fantastic image of a hippopotamus. This immediately felt like a message from the universe. I didn't have time to meditate on the meaning of it because I had to start writing this chapter, so I googled it. What I found from Imelda at trustedpsychicmediums.com was "The hippopotamus Spirit Animal reminds you that you are born great, and you have the potential to become whoever you want to be." I can't help but believe this message is for you right now at this point in this book! So I invite you to join me and take a few minutes to breathe that into your heart. Born great, born great. Potential to become whoever you want to be. I would love to help you with that.

I did a weeklong meditation retreat by myself in my home during which I meditated eleven to fourteen hours a day. At the end, I was told I was a spiritual teacher. This message came to me in a profound way, and I discovered what my work on this earth was and what my soul's purpose was, and frankly, I was terrified. While on the retreat, I could feel the truth in it, but once back to my everyday life, this knowledge felt more and more like a ball and chain.

At that time, I left Victoria, Canada to pursue my childhood dream to study fashion design, and I did the retreat over Christmas break. When I went back to school, my passion for the program fell flat; I had all but completely lost interest.

I kept thinking, "Why am I doing this if I am a spiritual teacher?" It suddenly all felt so meaningless. Some of my classmates were interested in meditation, so I started teaching them. I burned the candle at three ends. I was doing a two-year fashion design diploma program in one year, a two-year program in Heart Rhythm Meditation at IAM University of the Heart, and taught meditation part-time. I took time off from the fashion design program to attend five-day retreats and two-week residencies. I attended extra retreats than expected, as the retreats just called to me so strongly.

I finished the fashion design program and received the "overall completion award" and did nothing with it. I started to look at how I could combine fashion and spirituality, and in the end, nothing felt right. I wasn't able to fully step into the role of spiritual teacher and ended up sick because of it. Western medicine made me sicker, so I was on my own. I worked intensely on the root and sacral chakras to give the support my throat chakra needed. It took me time to recover, but the more I stepped into that role, the healthier I became. Here I am now, helping others move through what I went through in a lot less time.

It's taken me a long time, but I am so grateful for my journey. My soul's purpose is to help people like you. I am still not perfect by any stretch, but the tools I developed, acquired, and perfected over the decades helped me heal my neck pain permanently and allowed me to finally pursue my soul's purpose as a spiritual teacher and healer. Whatever your soul's purpose is and even if you don't know what it is, I can help you take the steps you are ready for today.

Chapter 3:

Is This Book for *You*?

"Yesterday I was clever, so I wanted to change the world. Today I am wise, so I am changing myself."
—Rumi

I want to help you heal your neck pain, so you no longer suffer the way you have. My wish is that, through the practices in this book, you will release your neck pain once and for all and move forward in your life in ways you have only dreamed of.

I wish I understood, decades ago, all that contributed to my neck pain at a subconscious level. I now see that I had to learn it all the long and hard way so that I could share my discoveries with you. One of the biggest things I realized years ago was that I played small. I played small without even realizing it in more than one area of my life. Do you play small in any area of your life? I don't want to see you playing small anymore. I did so for *way* too long. Even when I realized how small I played, it took me a decade to step out of that behavior. I wrote this book so you don't have to suffer anymore. My neck pain was but a symptom of a much deeper suffering. I wasn't ready to face that until I was in my forties, but once I did, my life took a great turn for the better. Our pain is an expression of something inside us that wants to heal and is ready to heal.

I invite you to let this book take you on a journey – a journey of deep self-discovery, profound healing, and unimaginable empowerment. This just may be one of those books you want to read again and again and again.

Throughout this book, you will gain a deeper understanding of your neck pain and throat chakra issues. The pain is so obvious and takes no effort whatsoever to pay attention to it. It does, however, take effort to look deeper and to dare to uncover the emotional and spiritual root causes of that pain. Your neck pain is like a weed in your beautiful garden; it stands out and doesn't contribute to the beauty. There is so much out there that can help you cut out that weed, but the weed always comes back, disrupting the beauty of your garden. It is only when the effort is put into digging right down to the tip of the root that it can be fully extricated, never to return again. This book will give you the tools you need to help you release and heal your neck pain and ensure it never comes back in the same way. You may end up with another weed – a different neck pain in the future – but these tools will serve you to do the same thing, and removing the weed just gets easier and easier once you know how to do it.

I have developed a number of unique and powerful spiritual practices inspired by various modalities and paths that are designed to maximize the amount of healing one can do through meditation. I combined meditation, energy work, and my own Heart-Centered Shamanism to help you delve into a journey of self-discovery and healing. This book is designed for people who want to make some serious changes and are ready to commit to themselves to do some deep work and move forward.

You likely already know about the chakras, what they are, and maybe even how they operate. You have possibly already worked with the chakras. If you know nothing about the chakras, this book will cover the basics of all the chakras and how they are all connected. I will help you get intimate with your personal chakras. It is not designed to tell you specifically how your chakras are the same as everyone else's. Through working with many people, I discovered that the experience of the chakras can be somewhat different for everyone, so my goal is to help you gain a more personal understanding of your chakras and how to work with what exists uniquely in your chakras. Of course, this book will serve you even if you are not familiar with the chakras.

By reading this book, you will gain a deeper understanding of your neck pain and throat chakra issues. This is fundamental. If you don't know what it is all about and what contributes to it, how can you possibly heal your chakra issues completely? Through these practices, you will not only discover the root causes of your suffering, but you will also become your own personal energy healer and will heal those root causes. Will it be easy? Sometimes, yes, but often, this journey will be difficult. However, I will say that the more difficult the journey, the greater the positive results. This work is extremely worthwhile.

Through these exercises, you will learn how to create the safety required to do this kind of work. I will help you create a sense of safety within yourself and outside yourself, which I believe is absolutely fundamental in working through a process such as you will experience with this book. Over time, you will be introduced to beginner through advanced practices designed to help you heal at various levels, one step at a time. You will be provided with detailed, step-by-step, guided meditations and unique spiritual practices. The healing portion is followed by practices that are designed to pull out the inherent light and beauty within you, empowering you to be who you truly are and, better yet, to help you take steps in pursuing your soul's purpose, whether you know what that is or not. The beautiful and unique light within you is covered by the hurts of the past, conscious and unconscious. Once you heal this covering made up of wounds, your light will begin to shine. There are practices that help you shine even brighter, helping you get in touch with the personal power latent within you so that you can take the steps you have dreamed of to move forward in your life and become who you truly are.

The throat chakra is an expression of what is within us. When we cannot express what is in our hearts and our being clearly and authentically, the throat suffers, and we find it more and more difficult to create the lives we desire. Many of us aren't even totally aware of all that is in us and wants to be expressed, so how can we possibly express what we don't know? This book helps you make great discoveries about who you are and who you are not. Once you learn the basic practices and move onto healing the first four chakras, you will work intensely in the throat chakra, which will help you create the changes your heart so desires.

The goal is to help you move toward purpose, and the throat chakra is the expression of that. There will be no more hiding your greatness; you cannot access your purpose when wounds are covering it.

You will learn to be your own spiritual guide, discovering the required steps you need to take to move forward in a whole new way. You will create a roadmap for yourself of action steps that you will actually be able to implement and will encourage and support you in taking giant steps to move forward in your life as you have not been able to do up until now.

The process is designed so that you feel as safe and supported as possible so that you can create the you that you were born to be. This process begins in Chapter 4 with a deep commitment to yourself to show up and do the work, a commitment to yourself to heal your neck pain and move forward in your life. In Chapter 5, a foundation for change is created with meditation, using breathwork to become your own energy healer, and I have included some excellent stretches to help at the physical level.

It's so important that you feel safe, so in Chapter 6, the focus on helping you develop both internal and external safety and a deeper sense of trust. One of my goals is to help you become your own teacher. I believe the teacher is doing their job when they help the student become their own teacher.

In Chapter 7, we will learn more and more about the chakras not just in a general way but the where, what, and how of the chakras at a very personal level. We are all unique and so are our chakras. In Chapters 8 and 9, I will help you to become your own energy healer through the practices provided. You will access spiritual support and heal wounds of the past. The more healing we do, the brighter our throat chakras shine!

In Chapter 10, we will work with Light Beings and your own personal light. Closer to the end of the process in Chapter 11, we will work intensely on the throat chakra to help you heal further and begin to express your truth and power in ways you haven't previously. We will work with what I have named "Heart-Centered Shamanism" in Chapter 12, working with specific Spirit Animals or Power Animals to help you create the change that has been just waiting to happen. We will then focus on empowerment and surrendering to your greatness in Chapter 13. You will begin to gain clarity on why you are here and begin to take giant steps toward your purpose whether you know exactly what that is or not.

Let me help you heal your neck pain so you can change yourself and change your life!

Chapter 4:

Spiritual Dating to Commitment

"Commitment unlocks the doors of imagination, allows vision, and gives us the right stuff to turn our dreams into reality."

—James Womack

Yes, we are spiritual seekers and there is *so much* out there to choose from – so many paths, so many modalities, and a whole lot of spiritual teachers, coaches, mentors, and healers. We can do what I call "spiritual dating" for years and years, and it works well and serves us to a degree. Spiritual dating is, in many ways, similar to dating in relationships. We try out different spiritual teachers or different spiritual paths and never stick to just one. It can be a lot of fun, enticing, and bring us some joy and lots of good feelings. It's a bit of an adventure, as we never know exactly what is going to happen. It is fun to try new things and get to know new people. It keeps our interest because there is always something new, and we can work with many teachers at the same time.

This can work well for us for a short time or a long time, but how intimate can we get with five people if we are dating them all at one time in our lives? How deep can we take multiple relationships compared to focusing on just one special one? It is when we decide that one person pulls at our heart strings that we would like to go deeper with that one person. It is the same with spiritual teachers. The deeper we go with one teacher, the deeper we can move into ourselves. It is when we discover one person – one method, teacher, or healer – who gives us greater hope and faith than another and commit to that one teacher for a period of time that opens the door to greater and lasting change. We need to say "No" in order to say "Yes, I am ready to explore myself through this teacher." Does that mean we stop all previous practices? Not necessarily. It just means that for this time, we commit to learning through one teacher for a certain period of time.

Along with this will often come some fear, especially these days with online dating where there are a plethora of people just waiting to get to know you. Spiritual dating is not like years ago when we met our soulmate through a friend, acquaintance, or happenstance. No, today, we could date a new person every day of the week if we so desired, and we could work with a new spiritual teacher every day of the week if we wanted. Doing so could be a great deal of fun, but how sustainable would it be?

I have met numerous people, and was one myself, who went from one spiritual teacher or spiritual path to another, jumping from one self-help book to another and one meditation style to another. If we look at all of these as relationships, which they are, how well does it serve us? It gives us new skills, new perspectives, experiences, thoughts, beliefs, practices, and new ways of being, but what would happen if we just chose one and made the commitment required to go deeper?

When we commit to the relationship with that one method or teacher in our hearts, we know that this person is the right one for us or the relationship is at least worth exploring. We can look him or her in the eye and say, "Yes, you are the one for me right now." How deeply can we make that commitment? It doesn't have to be a forever commitment; instead, it can be a commitment for a designated period of time like the time it takes to read this book. Essentially, the commitment is ultimately to yourself.

It's exciting to make this commitment and is often something worth celebrating, whether we celebrate outwardly or whether we celebrate within our hearts. It feels like a new beginning filled with hope, joy, and faith. We know we have made the right decision. Life is already better just by making this commitment. We can easily make the sacrifice of giving up spiritual dating and commit to this one teacher, path, or spiritual modality. There is a lift in our heels and in our heart. Everything is brighter, and it is through this commitment that we feel brighter and lighter. We are so open and hungry for what this teacher has to offer, knowing we will become more of who we truly are through the process of self-discovery, all the while deepening our connection with Source, God, or the Universe.

We feel hopeful, and our level of trust in life increases. We trust what we committed to, and that helps us trust ourselves and gives us faith that we will truly change for the better – until the inevitable happens and we are attracted to something else – to a new spiritual teacher – and we may just sneak away to listen to a talk, a podcast, or even a guided meditation. It may provide us with a fantastic experience, and we begin to wonder, "Oh no, did I make the wrong choice? Is this other person better for me? Have I made a terrible mistake? Well, I'm not too far into it, so maybe it's not too late to switch."

This frequently happens after making a commitment, and just know that this is the Universe's way of asking us, "Are you serious about this? Are you ready to take this plunge? Can you hold to your word?"

Have you ever been single for a long time, and then you meet someone and find yourself falling for them? This person seems perfect for you, like your souls were finally brought together as they were meant to be. Then, suddenly, out of the blue, other attractive people start showing an interest in you. You wonder, "How can this be? I was single for so long, and here I am, a magnet for love." This is how the energy of love works; it attracts more of the same. Therefore, when we commit to a spiritual process, method, or teacher, the same phenomenon occurs. The energy our hearts transmit will be reflected back to us. It's what we do with this that matters. We can take it as a cue to continue with spiritual dating, which we can do for the rest of our lives, or we can view it as a reflection of the magnified heart energy that is a result of this commitment, and we choose to stay with the one we chose.

I recommend focusing on this one spiritual process during the program this book offers and not starting a new spiritual path or skill until you have completed it. Yes, you may have a meditation practice already, but I suggest, for the time being, to just stick to what is offered here. If you are currently doing a meditation practice that you absolutely do not want to put on hold, you can certainly contact me to see how we can make it fit. Just send me a message at cherylstelte.com.

Commitment to Self

What about the commitment to self? Isn't this the most important of all? I certainly believe it is. We commit to the self when we commit to a relationship, and we commit to the self when we want to heal and grow. This can certainly exist in the path of spiritual dating or spiritual commitment.

I came to a point where I realized I'd been playing small my entire life. I subconsciously learned this behavior from my beloved father, and I desperately needed to move beyond it. I wondered how I managed that far, accomplishing a fair bit with the subconscious belief that if I played too big, I would get rejected or nobody would like me. Only if I played small would I be accepted. "Let others be bigger; let others shine brightly," I thought. "If I don't, I will be thought of as conceited."

My dad did his very best as a father. I think he thought his job was to keep us in line. I don't have any memories of my father ever giving me a compliment or saying anything kind. The first time I heard "I love you" from him was when I was twenty-eight. I had moved to another city, in another province, and at the end of a phone conversation, I said, "I love you," and he said, "I love you too." I will remember that forever. Again, I see this in some ways as a sign of the times. Did his father say kind words to him? I don't know. Was I loved? Yes. But the expression of love was repressed, and this caused me to have issues with unworthiness and not being good enough.

I grew up with the saying, "Always think of others before yourself." This was repeated to me by my mother. But I remember getting a plaque from my father that made me cry when I read all the words on it: "Fill your own cup first, and others will benefit from the overflow." I read that line over and over, and it slowly began to replace the old, worn-out belief of always putting others first.

It was quite a shock to receive such a gift from my father, whether he actually purchased it or not (I was pretty sure my future stepmother purchased it on his behalf). It felt like it was his way of making amends with me, and I still feel so much gratitude when I think of it. To this day, like many parents, I still believe in putting the children first, and I get great joy out of putting my adult children first. However, I make sure to always take good care of myself and my needs. When I received the plaque, I made a commitment to myself that I wanted a different life for myself, and I was going to do what I could to make the changes I desired. It was that the deep desire in my heart for change that brought me to start meditating.

I was thirty-two when I ended my marriage, and that was three weeks after one of my brothers ended his marriage. That same brother, who left his wife, committed suicide, which was something I think none of us thought we would ever get through. You don't know the pain of suicide unless you have gone through it, and I experienced a fair bit of guilt in thinking I could have done more to save my brother. That experience was the hardest thing my family ever went through together, and it still hurts today.

About six months after my brother's death, his spirit showed up on the beach at Deep Bay on Vancouver Island where a friend was doing kinesiology on me. We were at the beach waiting for the tide to go out so we could pick oysters. Picking oysters was on the top of my list of favorite things to do, and I love standing in the cold water, finding, gathering, and shucking oysters, and eating them raw.

As I laid on the beach and my friend plowed through different people and events in my life, I suddenly felt a great ball of love and light above me. I never experienced anything like it in my entire life, and I knew it was my deceased brother, Brian. I felt all this intense love. He was just love and light. Up until that point in my life, the extent of my spirituality had been going to church, which I hadn't done for years. My friend had never channeled before, and she didn't know I had a deceased brother. I didn't want to interrupt her flow but hoped she would mention him, and she did.

My friend said, "He is here."

I responded, "I know!"

Brian spoke through my friend, and we were both in awe as time stood still. We had a conversation around his death, and she told me that he was bipolar, and it was never diagnosed. He had gone to the light and was doing what he could, as spirit, to help people who were depressed or bipolar.

Then, I asked him why he was there. Brian said he wanted me to start to meditate. At that point, I would have done anything he said. I had heard of meditation but, at that point, had never tried it. By the next day, I was able to communicate with Brian myself. As we picked oysters the second day, I felt where he was and could hear him. It was such an uplifting and profound experience. By the time I got back to the city, the communication ended, and by the next day, I began to seriously question what happened. Was it real? Did I somehow make it up? Was it all fantasy?

However, even when the doubt came up, I started calling meditation places, and they all asked why I wanted to learn to meditate. I responded with, "So I can speak with my deceased brother," and they all informed me that they didn't have that kind of meditation. I was so disappointed! I knew nothing of the spiritual world and expected these people to understand.

At lunch that day, I went for a massage since I was recovering from a pinched nerve in my neck. When I walked down the hall to the office, I noticed a sign that said, "Meditation Classes," and the classes started the following evening. I signed up, went, and have been meditating ever since.

I made the commitment to myself to grow and live a better life, and the Universe responded by means of my beloved, deceased brother. I had no idea what I was getting myself into, but I had been on antidepressants myself for over a year and was able to get off them through meditation and never needed to go back on the medication. I made the commitment to myself then and never stopped. I never wanted to go back to the person I was, who was generally fairly unhappy and who didn't make the best choices for herself. I wanted to make better choices, and I longed for the happiness that I didn't have. I committed to meditating every day, starting with ten minutes. It wasn't until eight months later when I was up to meditating for twenty to thirty minutes that for the first time, I felt something significant. I felt different for less than thirty seconds. I didn't know what it was and couldn't describe it, but it was noticeably different. The feeling gave me the motivation to keep going. Over the decades, the Universe responded to my commitment to self and personal and spiritual growth in a variety of ways, and I am eternally grateful.

You are more than ready to make this kind of commitment if you haven't already. I invite you to look at what kinds of commitments you made to yourself over the years and how they served you. What kind of commitment are you ready for now? If you are reading this, you are more than ready to make a commitment to yourself; you just need to define it. What exactly are you ready for? How much change are you ready for? Are you tired enough of the pain in your neck and shoulders?

You have an understanding of throat chakra issues and recognize how your throat chakra holds you back. But are you ready to let go of your old ways of being and commit to something new? Are you ready to move beyond all you knew about yourself and enter into a journey of awakening to the real, more accurate you? This book was brought to you as an answer to your heart's call – your call for change. This is your call for a deeper understanding and knowledge of who you truly are so you can more fully express that in the world. Are you ready to make the commitment to yourself for deep, inner change so that you can create the outer change you so desire? Feel this in your heart right now.

See if you can breathe in the knowledge that all is happening exactly as it should, and you are ready. You are ready to make the commitment to yourself and the teachings in this book. It is time for you to change, to let go of the old, and invite in the new. If this doesn't resonate with you, I encourage you to pass this book to someone else. If you are emotionally moved by these words and feel a sense of hope or optimism, I invite you to keep reading. Often, we feel fear when we face the truth of what is in our hearts. So if you feel any fear or resistance to continuing to read this book – please – do yourself a huge favor and keep reading!

You are worth it; I'm just going to repeat that – *you are worth it*! You are worthy of all the blessings of the universe and to have a wonderful and fulfilling life. Yes, we will always have struggles, but living a full and fulfilling life is about the balance to be tipped toward joy and happiness, even with the struggles. I haven't met anyone who, once they look deeply, has not struggled with unworthiness. This is one of the main subconscious beliefs that holds us back from developing our full potential. The unworthiness is often developed in early childhood and serves us in our challenge to grow and become who we truly are, and we are worthy of that.

In this book, you will discover the best possible ways to move beyond fear and unworthiness, but for now, when you feel any uncomfortable feelings while you read through, please breathe deeply and allow yourself to feel any and all emotions fully. The heart wants to feel; it wants to feel everything, not just the positive, happy emotions but the most difficult emotions and everything in between. Can you make a commitment to yourself to feel your emotions fully? Trust me, this big commitment will serve you in lightening your load and allowing you to experience the positive emotions in ways you have not imagined.

Please take a bit of time here and reflect on what kind of commitment you are ready to make to yourself, to this book, or to me, as a teacher. I encourage you to read through before you make a big commitment to work with me, but for now, commit to reading this book, taking in the information and processing it to the best of your ability. This change doesn't have to take years either.

Commitment Meditation

I would like to guide you in a meditation to explore what your heart desires to help you discover what kind of commitment, if any, you are ready for. Are you ready to make a commitment to look at your throat chakra and heal all that you can? Are you ready to commit to expressing yourself in the best ways only your heart knows you can? Please follow me in this meditation.

As a special gift for you, you can also go to
https://cherylstelte.com/meditation/
to access some of the meditations in this book for free.

I invite you to sit in a chair where your feet are flat on the floor and your spine is very straight. Lift your shoulders up toward your ears and roll them back, letting them fall. You feel how this opens the chest, giving greater access to the heart center. Feel your seat in the chair and your hands in your lap, palms up or down – whichever is more comfortable.

I invite you to breathe deeply into the lower part of your abdomen, a long and full breath, stretching the length of the breath as long as possible, keeping your attention there for a few minutes. It helps to place your hand over your lower abdomen, with the thumb at the navel to keep your focus there, and breathe as low and deep as possible. When this begins to feel comfortable, place your hand on your heart center, and while breathing fully, bring your awareness to your heart center, which is in the middle of your chest.

Allow yourself to become aware of any thoughts or emotions that have arisen from reading this book so far. Just notice them, allow yourself to be with them, not wanting to push anything away. We want to allow everything the heart presents. We just keep breathing fully and noticing – noticing, feeling, allowing. Is there excitement, joy, hope, trust, faith, or wonder? Is there fear, resistance, longing, sadness, grief, hopelessness? Please allow yourself to feel whatever comes up without judgement.

You have come to a pivotal point in your life. You are ready for change, whether it is through this book, my program, or something else. You would not have purchased this book if you weren't ready for something. The best way to make a decision is to allow yourself to feel all that your heart wants and needs to feel. Our society does not encourage us to feel our feelings but instead, usually, to stuff them down. This is a great opportunity to sit and just be with yourself exactly as you are. Allow the emotions, even if you begin to cry. I have learned through the spiritual school, IAM Heart, that tears wash the heart, so at the very least, you will feel lighter after this meditation. Give yourself all the time you need to feel your feelings. If they change from happy to sad or vice versa, just allow that. Let your mind flow with the emotions of the heart.

Eventually, once you have felt all the emotions present in your heart at this time, notice what comes. Your heart has an inner sense of knowing; this is not the knowing of the mind. Just sit and focus on your heart and wait; wait for the knowing to appear. This inner knowing in the heart will let you know if it is best for you to commit to yourself in a new way and how. It will let you know if this is the book for you, if I am the person you are more than ready to work with, if you are ready to take the risk and learn new things so that you can grow and really let yourself shine.

This inner knowing may show up as thoughts, emotions, images, or body sensations, and, however obscure it may be, you will definitely recognize the sign(s). You already know if this is right for you or not. You will know if you have had enough of living the way you have been living and are open and willing to move forward into the unknown so that you may fulfill your heart's desires. You can easily access the longing in your heart and have the courage to sit with all that comes up. Change is never all that easy, especially great change. Small change can prove to be fairly easy, but the bigger the change, the more discomfort. Are you ready to get uncomfortable? I can promise you the temporary discomforts you will experience will always prove worthwhile, as they move us beyond our current discomfort of feeling stuck.

Are you ready to work with someone who always has your best interest at heart? Are you ready to work with someone who wants, more than anything, to see you shine in your most glorious and magnificent ways? What kind of commitment are you ready to make? Let your heart tell you. Let yourself feel your heart's desire fully, giving yourself all the time you need, and when you are ready, open your eyes.

Confident in Commitment

Congratulations on taking this crucial step and completing the meditation. Once you feel the kind of commitment you are ready for, it is beneficial to put it on paper and write it up in a journal. I recommend using a journal throughout this book beginning with this commitment so you can continue to look back on it, even recommitting when needed. This commitment holds us to it and helps us along when we experience regret or self-doubt, or the journey just gets hard. You may make a commitment to finish this program, and that is *a lot*! Your heart may already know that I am the person you want to work with based on what you have read to this point. You are open and ready for whatever it is I am going to offer and welcome the unknown. Now is the time to *begin* and put on paper the level of commitment that feels perfect for you in the face of your smaller self. Your true self knows. What is it that you can write down and sign today?

Here is a sample start, and I feel that it is important that you write the words for yourself. Please take your journal out and write it there or sit at your computer right now and write down whatever comes in your own, perfect words. For example, you might write, "I am so ready and willing to make the commitment to myself to heal my chronic neck and shoulder pain. It has been long enough, and I know I have lots of throat chakra issues. I am ready to face the sadness and disappointment that I feel, as well as this feeling of being stuck and the fear to move forward. I commit to this process with Cheryl Stelte. I commit to work with her the best I can. I commit to letting myself shine in ways I have never shone before. I commit to moving beyond my old ways and discovering my own inner beauty and uniqueness that will radiate out in the world so that I too may help others and be of service in ways I haven't even dreamed possible. Now is the time. I will commit to this process and welcome everything that comes. I welcome this journey of self-discovery so I can learn who I truly am and allow myself to move forward and express all that I have always meant to express. I sign my name here today."

Please read your commitment letter back to yourself, and listen to yourself as the receiver of the commitment. You are committing to yourself, so you are both the expresser of that commitment and the receiver. You can even meditate on receiving the commitment from yourself. Most people have a very different and often profound experience in being the receiver of their commitment to self.

Doesn't that just feel like a breath of fresh air? This is the first step and a very important one. I strongly encourage you to let yourself dive into this process with me. Know that I am already holding you in my heart every step of the way. Now that you feel confident in commitment, we can move onto the next step of creating a stronger foundation for change. You have already given yourself a sense of greater stability for the work of healing your neck issues, and we will take this one step further in the next chapter using meditation, breathwork and simple exercise.

Chapter 5:

Creating Safety

"Out of this nettle, danger, we pluck this flower, safety."
—William Shakespeare

I cannot emphasize enough the importance of safety when doing an intensive program such as this. How many times in your life have you felt unsafe? How many times have people said or done things to you that hurt so much, and you felt so unsafe in your fear and pain that you had nowhere to go? When we are abused, neglected, treated badly, ignored, criticized, yelled at, or ridiculed, we need to have a safety zone of some sort to offer us reprieve. Many of us grew up not knowing what that meant. Did you have the blessing of a parent who frequently said, "You can come to me with anything; I will always be there for you no matter what. You are safe with me?"

If you are reading this book, the likelihood is slim, and as I didn't, my parents didn't receive those words, nor did they have the wherewithal to say them or repeat those words when I needed to hear them most. How many of our parents, if they could do it all over again, would be our safety nets no matter what?

When I was a kid, we got food, clothing, and shelter, some fun summer vacations, and we even got to go out to restaurants once in a while. We played board games and cards as a family, but nobody talked about their feelings, especially feelings like fear, sadness, regret, joy, anger, etc. In fact, I don't know of too many families who did. It just wasn't the thing to do.

We expressed anger in our house by yelling, so I married someone who yelled a lot, and I hated it. I yelled too, and I hated it. Yelling doesn't create safety. I used to have conversations with a friend whose family didn't express anything – not anger, joy, or anything – nor did they talk about their feelings. Her mother left when she was young, and it was never talked about – not once. What is your story around expressing emotions and feeling safe?

In all the work that I do, one of my goals is to help people feel safe to move through the process this book provides. When I am doing energy healing, I let clients know that I am with them, they are not alone, they are safe, and it is okay to feel the emotions that move through them. My intention is to create a sense of safety for you as you read and do the work in this book.

Safety in Meditation Space

It is ideal to create a meditation space where you will not be disturbed. You want to create a sacred space in your home where you can sit on a chair and meditate. If you already have a daily rhythm and the perfect place in your home to meditate, you are set. If you have yet to develop a regular practice, you want to choose a place in your home where you will be undisturbed and where you can meditate at the same time every day, if your schedule permits.

First, you will need a comfortable chair. This is not the type of meditation where you sit on the floor for long periods and try not to move, even if your leg falls asleep or your shoulder is killing you. You want to be comfortable so you can focus your attention on your practices. If your nose gets itchy, please scratch it and keep meditating.

It's also ideal to meditate at the same time every day. I suggest mornings, as we are more awake and usually have more energy. For over five years after starting to meditate, I could not meditate in the mornings, as I was not a morning person. Instead, I meditated when I got home from work before I did anything else. Now, and for the last twenty years, I love meditating in the morning. Meditating in the evening can be challenging if you are tired. We need energy to do these practices, as they require concentration.

Look around for the best possible place – a corner of a room is perfect – and ask yourself if it is a safe-feeling space. Will you be able to cry if need be and not worry about being judged by another person walking by at the time you do the practices? Maybe you live with other people and none of them would understand, or maybe they would support you. In any case, it likely needs to be a private space where you can be alone with yourself. Take some time to sit in your sacred space. How safe does it feel on a scale of one to ten?

We are aiming for an eight at least. At the same time, if you do not feel safe anywhere on earth, it's totally fine if you don't get the eight. If the rating is lower than that, you need to make whatever changes you can think of so that you feel very safe in your physical meditation space. Try to think of what might be missing, what would help your space feel more comfortable and safe – it might even be a favorite scarf that you love to wear.

Please sit in your space and imagine what would help you feel safer. If there is no way you can have visible privacy, maybe you want to hang a curtain or put a room divider around your space, or maybe you need to change your space to another area of your home. Maybe there is only one time in the day where you can be there alone and that is the time when you will feel most safe. If such a time does not exist, you can ask the person living with you if they can alter their schedule a bit so that you can have a bit of alone time if there is not a physical room you can go to. Freedom to sit with whatever comes up in this book will help you move beyond your blocks and what is holding you back in life.

Once you feel you have the privacy you need, are there any pictures or objects that always give you a good feeling when you look at them or touch them? These could be crystals, statues, lighting, plants, flowers, wall hangings, or photos of your grandmother or grandfather, spiritual guru, goddess, loved one(s), nature scenes, animals, birds, or whatever makes you feel good, possibly even supported, and especially safe.

What is on the floor of your space? Do you want to put a little area rug to sink your toes into or do you love the natural feel of wood? How comfortable is your chair? Does your back get sore after meditating a while? Do you need to have a cushion nearby to slip behind it to support it so you can continue meditating?

Please put some effort into refining your space so that you experience a sense of safety when you sit there. If any of the aforementioned helps you feel supported as well, please make sure to incorporate that. You can never have too much support. Once completed, confirm with yourself that the sense of external safety is at a level of an eight or the greatest level you can create, given what you have to work with. If you just can't seem to get to a level of safety you enjoy, it may be that your internal sense of safety is just so low that all the external safety in the world will not make you feel safe. You need to go inside and start to create safety internally. We will do that in this chapter.

Internal Safety

Carl Jung, founder of analytical psychology, taught about the inner child – the child who has repressed emotions, unmet needs, unhelpful core beliefs, deep seated fears, etc. This inner child usually didn't experience a strong sense of safety. Many people, including me, believe that our souls choose our parents. Hazrat Inayat Khan, a great Sufi master, wrote about the soul coming from the angelic planes. He taught that souls are like the rays of the sun, some long and some short. The long rays are souls that have come down to earth and have a unique purpose to accomplish as a human being. We are all one of those long rays. The thing with becoming human is that the soul is ready and agrees to face the human challenges, forgetting itself as the angel in bliss. Your soul came into this life agreeing to engage in the struggle of humanity as a human being, and that began when you were born or possibly even in the womb. It is extremely beneficial for our work on earth to heal the wounds of the past so that we can shine the light we came in with. Each one of us has something unique and important to accomplish. It's never easy for anyone, and if your inner child does not feel safe because of events – familial, environment, and circumstances – it is ideal to help her/him feel safe.

Fifty or one hundred years ago, I don't think you would have heard people say what many people say today, "I am in my head; I'm not centered. I'm not grounded; I was out of my body." Many of us now know that we will feel better and safe if we feel centered and grounded. I'm sure you know some grounding exercises, or at least one. The one I practiced for years was imagining and sending a grounding cord from the root center down into the earth, even all the way to the center of the earth. This is very useful, and I would like to take this a few steps further.

Creating Safety Meditation

I invite you to sit in the meditative posture with your spine very straight. The spine is a transmitter and receiver of energy, so you want to make the most of it by sitting very straight yet relaxed. Bring your awareness to the spine, following it up and down, feet on the floor and hands in the lap, with palms facing down, roll the shoulders up and back, giving them a nice stretch as you do that. Bring your aware-ness to the heart center and take on the full breath, engaging the abdominal muscles to help expel all the air on the exhale and inhale fully and completely while you let the belly expand.

Once you are comfortable with the full breath, find the heartbeat and make the breath rhythmic with an eight/eight count, more or less being fine too. After breathing this way for five to ten minutes or until it feels natural and easy, continue the rhythmic breath and imagine you have a grounding cord that goes from your lower torso down into the earth. Imagine what color and texture it is or if it has a temperature.

If you do not see or imagine anything, notice if you feel any sensations or have a sense of knowing the grounding cord is there. Once you are in tune with your grounding cord, I invite you to exhale ener-gy from your heart down into the earth, creating a strong connection with the earth. On the inhale, breathe up the unconditional love of mother earth into your heart center. Breathe and direct the heart's energy in this fashion for a few breaths, and then widen it. Imagine that when you exhale, the stream of energy becomes wider, making the grounding cord wider and wider until it reaches the earth and goes straight down. We inhale up that wider stream of en-ergy into the heart center. Every exhale, we widen the cord a little more so we can exhale more heart energy and inhale more heart energy. We keep breathing this way until the grounding cord from the heart includes our legs out to our knees and our feet are entirely in the grounding cord. It may feel like a pyramid shape or even like an umbrella, but our connection with the earth is very wide.

Feel how stable you feel with a such a wide connection. See if you can feel your heart energy going down and running through your legs, feet, and the space around you. Then fill that space with unconditional love from mother earth. Continue with this practice until you feel solid, stable, and safe.

Next, imagine yourself as a small child. What age are you? Can you see or feel what you are wearing? Where are you? What are you feeling? How safe in the world do you feel? What doesn't feel safe? Who doesn't feel safe? I invite yourself to look at or feel your feet as that small child. What are you wearing on your feet? How do your feet feel in those socks, shoes, boots, or whatever is there? How grounded do your feet feel? How safe do you feel with what's on your feet? This is an opportunity to help your inner child feel safe and grounded. Please take the time to change the footwear on your inner child, taking off what exists and putting on what you know would be perfect for him/her to have fun, feel safe, and feel grounded. Take your time. You may need to try on a few different items. What color would you make the footwear? How does it feel? How does the little child in you feel with the new footwear? Hold the little you in your heart and let your inner child know you will keep him/her safe and grounded. You will be there for your inner child always, keeping him/her safe. Let your inner child know that you will be back to hold him/her again very soon and will continue to hold them in future. Give yourself time to really connect and love the little you, and when it feels right, open your eyes.

How was that meditation for you? Write down your experiences in your journal. Maybe the little you had something to say for you to write down as well. You can repeat this meditation any time or as often as you wish. It's not about getting it right or wrong; it's about the experience and making the inner child feel safe.

Often, your sense of trust in the self and trust in the Universe is based in your sense of safety or lack of a sense of safety in your inner child. My wish and intention is to help you reach a new level of trust – to trust more deeply in yourself and your capacity to expand your sense of trust in the Universe and Source and that you are here for a unique and glorious reason specific to only you and to help you trust in this process of healing and empowerment. Deepening your trust leads to faith and living with trust and faith will make a difference, even in your daily existence.

Safety in What or Who Is Presented

I remember when I met Claude Poncelet for the first time at a three-day shamanism workshop. He is an amazing, self-

52

taught shaman from Belgium. I felt like I had found my spiritual teacher and spiritual family. I travelled from Victoria, British Columbia, Canada to a rustic retreat center south of Seattle with a friend. I remember feeling at home with all these strangers. Claude led us on a spiritual shamanic journey to invite in the Power Animal that wanted to work with us that weekend, and we explored our connection with Power Animals and what they came to teach us.

Power Animals, Totem Animals, or Spirit Animals usually refer to the essence of that animal in general. All animals have distinct qualities and each animal has a unique essence. When we connect or take on a Power Animal, we are not connecting with an individual animal but to the essence of all of that specific species on the planet. For example, the gorilla was one of my first Power Animals, and it was male. The male gorillas do an amazing job of protecting their entire families, and it was beneficial for me to feel protected and safe.

During that workshop, a new Power Animal showed up immediately for me, and it was the elephant. Not an actual elephant, but the general spirit of all elephants came to me in order to help me grow or develop in some way. I was so surprised, but soon after working with the elephant, I began to slow down to a pace I was unaccustomed. I was going so fast in my life, working long hours at my then business, Stelte Design, and living a very busy life, living way too fast. This was exactly the spiritual medicine I needed in my life at that time.

Years later, when I sacrificed shamanism in order to commit to HRM and my new teachers, Susanna and Puran Bair, I remember meditating once and suddenly realizing that somehow Susanna Bair called me. There was a calling I responded to. This was not something I knew previously, but that day I knew I was in the right place at the right time.

I invite you to reflect on how this book came to you. I encourage you to take out your journal or a piece of paper and write down what comes to you when you think of the following questions: How did you hear about me? Why are you reading this book? How do the few practices feel so far? How do you relate to the stories? What were you wishing for or dreaming of before you discovered this book? What are your biggest hopes? What has your spiritual journey been like until now? What would you like your spiritual journey to be like? What do you know needs to change the most or first?

Additionally, ask yourself what you tried before to get rid of your neck pain? How tired are you of having a stiff and sore neck? How long have you had throat chakra issues? How do you know this book is right or wrong for you? What are you feeling about this book right now? Are you ready for a change? How ready are you to face the inevitable discomfort that true and lasting change brings? Here is a meditation to help you go from the mind and into your heart for deeper knowing on these questions. This is to help you get clarity around whether this is the right book for you or not.

Clarity Meditation

Get into the posture, taking your time to feel your body sit nice, and straight, and strong while relaxed. Breathe into your heart center and begin counting the heartbeats. Breathing into and out of your heart, ask your heart what your level of trust in this book is. Nobody can answer this question except you. Go straight into the center of your heart center. The heart chakra is located along the spine and not in the front of the chest, so breathe closer to the back of the body, as this also helps you go deeper. Ask yourself, what is my level of trust that reading this book is very good for me, or something similar? Is this book a blessing for me or not? Without knowing what is in this book yet, how does your heart feel about continuing to read it? If it's time to pass the book on, that is fine! This is about you and what is best for you. Explore whatever you notice or feel in your heart. Is there a sense of knowing of sorts? What exists in your heart around this book?

If you ever feel sleepy practicing HRM, it's usually because your breath is not full enough. I still check in with my abdomen occasionally to make sure I am breathing fully. The practices have a greater effect when you breathe as fully as possible. It may feel like a bit of a workout in the beginning, but you get used to it.

If you have been doing another style of meditation, I encourage you to just try this method for a while and see how it fits. Do it as an experiment for a month or two, and if you don't like it, go back to your old method. Please feel free to contact me at cherylstelte.com to ask any questions.

My hope here is that you have clarity around if you are meant to read this book and do the program contained therein on your own or with me personally. It will benefit you to be aware of your level of safety and trust moving forward. It doesn't have to be perfect, and you can even feel a certain amount of unsafety and little trust and read the book. The more aware you are, the better for you. This is a great practice for anything we want to embark on. Sometimes our minds find something enticing but it is short-lived. Getting in touch with our level of safety and trust with anything helps us make the commitment to ourselves if that is what's best for us. Spiritual dating is a great thing, and when we are ready to go deeper, making commitment to one thing, even if for a designated period of time, such as eleven weeks, it is most beneficial to create the change your heart longs for.

I hope you have found a new sense of deep safety within and without yourself to trust and do the practices in this book to continue on this journey of self-discovery, healing, and empowerment. Know that you can come back to this chapter at any time if you start to get uncomfortable with anything that comes up for you. This is your safe haven chapter.

We have begun to create a foundation for change through creating a deep sense of safety to do this work. In the next chapter, we will continue with developing through other techniques.

Chapter 6:

Creating the Foundation for Change with Meditation, Breathwork, and Simple Exercise

"Spirituality is in no way a hindrance to worldly progress. A worldly success when gained through the power of spirituality has a stronger foundation."

—Hazrat Inayat Khan

In order to manifest the changes you deeply desire, you need to first create a strong foundation, one that will support you through all the highs and lows of this process. You want to be at your fundamental best physically, mentally, energetically, and spiritually. You do not need to be a superstar, but you need to start with as solid a foundation as possible, and that means, for most of us, a notch or two above where you are currently.

Physically, I understand most of you who are reading this book are currently experiencing a certain level of pain, likely in the neck and/or shoulders. My goal is to help you ease into this a certain amount, and I will share with you some of my favorite exercises that get results without having to spend one hour a day doing yoga or other stretching exercises. Fifteen minutes will do the trick. This will create a physical foundation for the work ahead. Mentally, you will just read your commitment to self every day as a reminder of what you are doing and why you are doing it. Energetically, you will discover the power of breath and learn to direct it. This is the foundation for becoming your own energy healer and will help you dive into that work in future chapters. Spiritually, we will cover the basics of the Full Rhythmic Breath, which will give you an amazing foundation for spiritual growth and change.

Exercises to Ease Neck Pain

Let's start with the physical aspect. I'm sure you have tried various forms of western medicine, alternative therapies, and treatments to heal your neck pain. Some of them have helped and some not, but even if something(s) helped, the same pain keeps coming back, or it returns in a different way. Nothing you tried helped you eliminate your neck pain entirely. I would like to share some of the exercises that helped me tremendously.

As you know, I had a pinched nerve in my neck, and it took a great deal of time to recover from that, having suffered with intense pain for over eighteen months. The number one stretching exercise that helped me is a bit of a spinal twist and what I refer to as the cross-over stretch.

Cross-Over Stretch

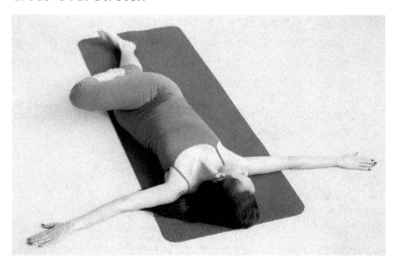

- Lie down on your back on the floor or a yoga mat and raise your knees.

- Put your arms out to your sides at a ninety-degree angle from the body, with palms facing down.

- Lift your right leg and cross it over your left leg, letting both legs fall to the left, without letting your right shoulder come off the floor.

- Keeping your shoulders on the floor and your hands face down, turn your head to the right as far as possible without making you uncomfortable.

- It is important to not push to a level of pain during this stretch. Try to breathe as deeply as possible, and with each breath, relax the body, letting it fall to the floor. I like to count seconds and, depending on your level of flexibility and current pain, allow yourself to remain in the stretch for thirty to ninety seconds before repeating it on the other side. I found the best time for me to do this stretch is in the late evening before bed. It helps me relax so I can easily sleep as well as providing the best relief from neck or shoulder tension or pain.

- As you see in the image below, her shoulders are on the floor. Please do not let the shoulders rise from the floor as it may cause injury.

Acupressure

Once you are in bed, it is an ideal time to do a little acupressure on your neck. Acupressure is similar to acupuncture but uses human fingers instead of needles. It works with the meridians, which are energy pathways that run through our bodies. There are a number of pathways that run through the back of the neck, and by pressing certain points, we can release stuck energy and get that energy flowing more easily again.

I think the best time to do this is as soon as you get into bed. Get yourself comfortable in bed and have your room at your ideal level of warmth for sleep. Lie flat on your back and take a few long, deep breaths, focusing on the exhale; exhale with a sigh. This is an opportunity to let go of all the worries of the day and breathe in the regeneration we experience in sleep.

- Begin by applying finger pressure at the small intestine points behind the arm socket. To locate these points, cross your arms over your chest and reach around to your underarm on each side with your middle finger. Slowly slide your finger two to three inches up the space where the arm joins the body with slight pressure, looking for a tender spot. It is often halfway between the underarm and the top of the shoulder. There are actually a number of points along here. Feel around for a sensitive spot and apply pressure with one finger on each side. Press as hard as feels comfortable, and breathe deeply for about two minutes if you can; three minutes is a lot, and more is not always better.

- Next, put your arms down by your side and then lift your hands up and place two to three fingers on the shoulder points which are located by placing your fingers on the shoulder one to two inches away from your neck. You can also run your fingers along the top of your shoulders and find the most sensitive spot. Anyone reading this book will likely have tension in the shoulders, so press there for a couple minutes while breathing deeply into the lower abdomen.

- We then want to follow the remaining points up the neck and find our way up to the points at the base of the skull. Locate these points by placing a couple fingers on the spine at the neck and slide them outward slowly until you feel the muscles, about one and a half inches out. Apply pressure on each side of the neck at these points for as long as is comfortable.

• Alternate which fingers you use so they do not get sore. Find a balance between discomfort and relief. If your arms or fingers get tired, put them back down by your side and just breathe deeply and rest for a while. Resume what you are doing when it feels right.

• Please place your hands in front of you and bring your hands together, crossing and locking your fingers together. Keeping fingers locked together, bring your hands behind your head and use your thumbs to find the points at the base of the skull. Slowly slide your thumbs outward until you find where there is a natural indentation. Release the fingers and get comfortable. Press on these points at the base of the skull, pressing upward for as long as possible. This is the final release. This exercise will release some neck pain and provide some great relaxation as well as a great start to a good night's sleep.

We do need to move physically, as we are physical beings. If you have an exercise routine that works for you, keep doing it! As a minimum, I recommend yoga sun salutations. This was the most effective exercise for recovering from the pinched nerve in my neck. I am providing a point by point description here, and please also feel free to try out yoga if you haven't already. If your pain level is very high, there are all sorts of classes for people with back pain and these same instructors can usually help anyone with neck pain. Please let the image shown following the instructions be your guide and be patient with yourself. It took me some time to memorize the sequence, but once you do, you have it for life.

Hatha Yoga Sun Salutation

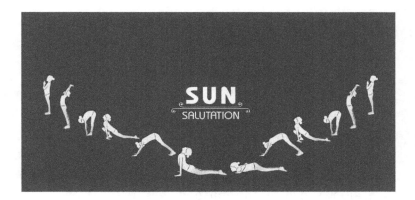

- Stand in one place with your feet together or two to three inches apart, big toes touching, heels out

- Press the palms lightly together in front of the chest with the shoulders back and down

- The crown of the head lifts up, and the chin is parallel to the floor

- Inhale and sweep the arms up and look up at the thumbs

- Lift out of the waist, reaching up towards the sky

- Exhale as you bend forward and down from the waist into forward fold

- Press the palms flat on the floor (or as far as you can get), bending knees slightly. Line fingertips up with toes

- Bring your forehead towards the legs

- Inhale and step the right foot back into a high lunge. Make sure the left knee is over the ankle and toes are pointing forward

- Shoulders are back and down, the chest presses forward, crown lifts up, and the back leg is straight

- Step the left foot back into a plank, so the body is one straight line and in a push-up position

- Press the heels back and reach the crown of the head forward

- Exhale bending the knees to the floor and bend the elbows to lower the chin and chest to the floor

- Reach the hips up towards the sky, arching the back. Inhale into upward facing dog, scooping the chest forward, straighten the arms, and roll onto the tops of the feet

- Reach the crown of the head up, press the chest forward, and lift the hips and legs off of the floor; bend the elbows slightly if it feels like you are straining the low back

- Exhale into downward facing dog, tucking the toes under, bend the elbows, and lift the hips up and back

- Press firmly into the hands and arms to press the hips back, letting the head hang from the neck press the heels into the floor. The legs are straight or can be slightly bent to flatten the back

- Inhale and step right forward into a high lunge, stepping the right foot forward between the two hands and adjusting the leg so that the knee is directly over the ankle and the toes and knee are pointing forward

- Keep the back leg straight as you sink the hips down; the crown lifts up, and the chest and gaze are forward

- Exhale into forward fold, pressing the palms flat to the floor; if necessary bend the knees slightly

- If you have the flexibility, bring the fingertips in line with the toes

- Reach the forehead in towards the legs and inhale and sweep the arms up

- Stay in Mountain alignment, and look up at the thumbs, lifting out of the waist, reaching up towards the sky

- Exhale and bring the palms together in mountain and place the feet together or two to three inches apart, parallel, and facing forward

- The palms are lightly pressed together with the shoulders back and down, and the chest presses in towards the thumbs while the crown of the head lifts up, and the chin is parallel to the floor

Depending on your current level, start with what feels easy and just push yourself a little further. For example, if doing three feels good and four sun salutations starts to feel hard, just do four and increase as you can, continuing every morning. Know that you are not only helping your neck; you are helping your entire body.

Meditation and Breath

You've heard the story about what motivated me to start meditating, and I must say, it is one thing that has provided me with the most healing and personal and spiritual growth. I am a different person today than I was twenty-five years ago. Yes, we all change, or at least most of us change over the years, but I am so grateful to have meditation to help me heal and grow to become the person I am today. I would never have even come close without it.

I started with a type of mindfulness meditation, read various books, and tried different methods. I worked with the chakras for years and eventually discovered shamanism. Meditation and shamanic practice are two different practices, and I did both for years. When I discovered Heart Rhythm Meditation, which was developed by Puran and Susanna Bair, my meditations went to a whole new level. This was soon after I had ended a very difficult relationship and went to India for four and a half months to recuperate and get my yoga teacher training. During that time, I did a lot of meditation on the third eye, staying at an ashram, and meditating a great deal, as part of the yoga teacher training. I was on a spiritual quest and loved the experiences of upward meditation.

Before that, I enjoyed meditating on my heart center and moving energy through all the chakras. When I returned from India, I missed meditating on my heart center, and while I tried to do my old meditations, I could not keep my energy there, no matter how hard I tried. My energy kept going up. Eventually, out of frustration, I googled "heart and meditation" and discovered HeartMath and Heart Rhythm Meditation. I found a couple of free meditations online and favored the Heart Rhythm Meditation, and I ordered Puran and Susanna's book, *Living from the Heart*.

As soon as the book arrived, I jumped right in and in little time was able to keep my energy and focus in my heart center. After a number of months of doing the practices every day, one day my heart center suddenly grew to be bigger than me; I was sitting inside my heart. This was so amazing for me. All I felt was this deep, pure love – nothing else. The room seemed brighter, and the love just flowed through me. The experience lasted about twenty to thirty minutes. I used to fall out of peak experiences if I thought certain thoughts, but this incredibly strong experience held and held. I just sat there and wept in the beauty of love as I breathed my enormous heart. It was like time stopped, and I became a being of light and love, fully here and present, but my physical self fell into the background.

I could still feel my heartbeat throughout the experience, but I was more in my energetic self than my physical self. It was like my soul came out of me and expanded, taking over. My soul is pure light and love, and that is simply what I was for that twenty to thirty minutes. When it subsided, I grabbed the book and went to their website, and after reading about their two-year intensive program, I signed up for IAM University of the Heart and did all of IAM Heart's trainings. I am now on the faculty, co-teaching graduate programs in addition to teaching and mentoring my own students. I am also a personal retreat guide.

In this book and in all my programs, we will be using the "Full Rhythmic Breath" which is the foundation practice of Heart Rhythm Meditation. The more advanced practices in this book were developed over time by spirit moving through me and guiding me. These practices have benefited myself and others immensely, and I look forward to sharing these with you in upcoming chapters. For now, we will begin with the Full Breath and then move onto the Full Rhythmic Breath (FRM).

Basic Full Breath Meditation

Posture is of importance to practice the Full Rhythmic Breath; sit on a comfortable chair with the spine straight and the head lifted toward the ceiling. The spine is our major energy highway, consisting of the chakras, or energy centers, which are located at the spine, along with the energy channels that run along the sides, the Ida and Pingala (this will be discussed further later). The main thing is that you want to keep the spine as straight as possible for optimum energy flow. Your feet are flat on the floor and about hip-width apart. You want the knees to be level with the hips, which allows you to breathe fully into the lower abdomen. The hands are placed on the thighs either palms up or down, whichever feels right to you. Palms up are more receptive and palms down are more grounding. We have chakras in the feet and hands and facing both downward and connecting to these chakras helps us become grounded and centered. I learned the value of keeping the spine straight early on, and it was IAM Heart where I learned to keep the level of the knees below the hips. IAM Heart calls this posture the Pharaoh posture. Once seated and comfortable, lift the shoulders up toward the ears and roll them back, letting them fall. Feel the opening of the chest and the heart center.

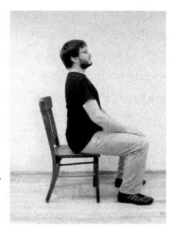

I want you to remember this: *breath is what powers the practices.* Without a full breath, you will not have the effect you desire. This is probably the hardest part to perfect, but the benefits are endless. Breathing with a full breath and engaging the abdominal muscles calms the nervous system and stimulates the vagus nerve, which transmits information to or from the surface of the brain to tissues and organs elsewhere in the body. This oxygenates the body and allows access to your subconscious.

No one ever exhales completely in their daily breathing due to a subconscious fear of death. If we exhale all the way, there will not be another breath and we will die. With the Full Rhythmic Breath, it is so important to exhale all the way and expel all the air completely. We exhale all that has been used up and subsequently invite in the new. Every breath is a new beginning, so at the end of the breath, you want to focus on how far you exhale. You want to give the abdominal muscles an extra little squeeze after you think you exhaled all the air, as there is usually just a little further you can go with this. The abdomen automatically wants to expand, and this is where we can breathe in new life on the inhale. It's exciting that we can take the time to prompt change in this way just through the breath.

> *Sitting in the posture described above, I invite you to place your hand on your lower abdomen with your thumb over your naval. Begin by taking long, deep breaths, doing your best to breathe into the lower abdomen. On the inhale, we fill up the lower abdomen like a balloon, breathing in as much as possible, while keeping the shoulders and the rest of the body relaxed. On the exhale, we squeeze the abdominal muscles to expel all the air.*

This takes some practice, as we are all used to breathing into our chest, or some of us are used to only breathing into our shoulders. Deep breathing takes times to learn, and I trust you will have patience with yourself. When we breathe fully in this way, brain function changes. In our everyday breath, the medulla oblongata at the back of the brain is in charge of breathing. As soon as we engage the abdominal muscles, that brain function moves to the frontal lobe brain and, in so doing, frees up the back of the brain. This freeing up of the back of the brain allows access to your subconscious.

In this style of meditation, the intention is not to get rid of thought. For years, I heard people say they couldn't meditate because they can't get rid of their thoughts. We value our thoughts when they come from the subconscious. Yes, you may still have thoughts about what to make for dinner or how we want to spend your weekend, but you have more and more to concentrate on, so it keeps the mind busy and those everyday thoughts are not so intrusive. You want to access the subconscious because it brings up your own internal guidance, memories of the past that want to be healed, and more and more information about who you truly are and how you can best pursue and live your purpose here on earth.

Full Rhythmic Breath

The last step is to find and focus on the heartbeat. You want to practice the above posture and breath until the full breath becomes automatic; otherwise, it can be difficult to focus on the heartbeat and breathing fully at the same time. Depending on how much breathwork you have done, this can take from one hour to three weeks. Focusing on the heartbeat helps you get in touch with your rhythm, which creates more rhythm in your life. How much out of rhythm is your life? This small step helps a great deal in helping you find your own internal rhythm, which reflects in your outer life.

Full Rhythmic Breath Meditation

Begin with the posture, and practice breathing fully until it feels natural or at least comfortable. Place the fingertips of one hand over the sternum in the center of the chest, applying a bit of pressure. Sit and breathe fully and notice if you can feel the heartbeat vibrating through the fingertips. Continue with that for a couple minutes. Next, try placing the flat of the hand or the flat of the fingers over the physical heart. Can you feel your heartbeat this way? The third method is to hold the breath after the inhale. Now, it's important that we don't hold the breath in the chest. Of course, when we are stressed, we hold the breath in the chest and tense our shoulders. This can be hard on the nervous system and hard on the organs. You want to keep the shoulders relaxed and hold the breath in the belly.

After the inhale, hold the breath for as long as is comfortable and then exhale. This is often a reliable way to feel the heart beating. It can take some time to feel the heartbeat, and if this is you, don't worry, it will come. Over the years spent teaching, I find that as we slowly move to becoming more heart-centered, more and more people find their heartbeat faster than they used to. Once you find your heartbeat or even your pulse, you want to count how many heartbeats you feel on the inhale and how many you have on the exhale. Over time, the goal is to get to eight heartbeats in and eight heartbeats out. Some of us start at four or six and others, and often athletes or those who have worked with the breath previously start with ten or twelve. The starting point doesn't matter so much as the fact that you feel something. The next step is to make the number of heartbeats on the inhale the same as the number on the exhale.

If you don't feel your heartbeat or pulse, no need to worry; you can count seconds. This is called the Full Rhythmic Breath. It is a long, full inhalation and long, full exhalation, breathing into the lower abdomen while you follow the rhythm of the heartbeat using six or eight counts in and six or eight counts out. Please practice this as long as you can.

Directing the Breath

With the Full Rhythmic Breath mastered, you can begin to direct the breath. This is how you will become your own energy worker. We are energetic beings, and we can make the most of this by learning to direct the breath in ways that heal and empower us. I can write about all the scientific proof about humans being energetic beings, but I would like you to experience your own energy in a simple and easy way. This practice is a Heart Rhythm Meditation practice.

Directing the Breath Meditation

Please sit in the Pharaoh posture and take on the Full Rhythmic Breath. When that is flowing nicely, find your heartbeat, and breathe with an eight count. Lift your dominant hand up so the palm is facing you. Open your eyes and place the center of your palm in front of the center of your chest and about six inches away. Close your eyes again, and focus again on the posture and full, rhythmic breath. You want to then see the intention that you will exhale

73

your heart's energy from your heart and through the palm of your hand in front of you. We are breathing fully with the belly in the background and focus on sending the heart's energy into the space in front of you through the hand. Keep doing this until you feel the physical sensations created in the center of the palm by the energy directed there. Just keep breathing in this fashion until you feel something. You might feel warmth or coolness, tingling, or even pulsing. You may need to do it for a while or even repeat the exercise a number of times, but you can do this. This exercise just helps the mind believe that you can, and will, direct energy.

I encourage you to practice the Full Rhythmic Breath every day for ten to twenty minutes to start and eventually over time sitting for forty-five minutes. That may sound like a lot, but most people spend the first twenty to thirty minutes on technique, and once we get over the thirty-minute hump, we feel the practice working for us energetically. It's in the last fifteen to twenty minutes where we get the energetic and emotional results. One of the biggest challenges is to develop a regular, daily practice. Once you are sitting, it's usually pretty easy. It's getting yourself to sit every day. This is where the personal commitment comes in. Maybe you want to read your commitment every morning when you get up. I find that the long-term goal is forty-five minutes. That may sound outrageous, but I find that most people quit at twenty minutes. This is when we get bored, or it's when our stuff or issues start to come up.

This reminds me of when I used to swim lengths. My son swam in a swim club for some time, and I admired all these kids whose bodies flowed so beautifully through the water. Eventually, I wanted to do the same thing and took an adult stroke correction course so I could swim multiple lengths. I discovered swimming is not just about the strokes but so much about how we breathe!

Swimming in a twenty-five-meter pool, the first three or four lengths were a piece of cake. However, it slowly became more difficult for me to continue. My muscles started to ache a bit. I doubted I could continue the breathing, and I started with the negative self-talk, such as, "Why am I even doing this? What was I thinking? This is so hard. I should just go home; today is not the day for this. I feel weak, etc."

This continued until I would get over the hump of the twelfth length; then everything changed. I got into the flow of swimming, and it became easy. I felt the joy of my body gliding through the water. I usually did 100 to 110 lengths in an hour even though I was a smoker. I enjoyed the swimming so much that I eventually quit smoking, and my lengths went up to 120.

Meditating is similar; it starts to get hard at twenty minutes, but if you can push through that next ten, you are over the hump and in the flow. Just keep breathing, and just keep counting heartbeats, as awkward or uncomfortable as it becomes. This is where you begin to have deep and profound experiences. Trust me, it is worth the effort. You won't get there overnight, and you definitely need to practice, but you just need to trust you will get there and keep sitting and practicing. Most of us can only meditate once a day, but in truth, meditating twice as day is optimal. After developing the ability to sit for forty-five minutes, I recommend forty-five minutes in the morning and ten to thirty minutes in the evening, especially when you are serious about change and/or are going through a program such as the one in this book. It is certainly not all bliss; healing happens in longer meditations, and that can be hard at times, but you will also move into the heights of joy and glorification!

You have learned how to create a great foundation for change with physical exercise, basic acupressure, breathwork, and the Full Rhythmic Breath. We will now be moving onto the chakras and your own personal discovery of their location and how you experience them. I will be holding you in my heart as you take these steps forward and begin to develop one of the practices that will help you become more of who you truly are.

Chapter 7:

Getting Intimate with Your Unique Chakras

"The soul is the divine breath. It purifies, revivifies, and heals the instrument through which it functions."

—Hazrat Inayat Khan

No doubt you know something about the chakras. You likely know they are energy centers that are located within our bodies and energetic beings. Today, whether I am teaching or healing, it amazes me how many people know about the chakras. It seems to me that twenty years ago, not many people did, nor were they interested. I'm grateful for your current knowledge and your openness to learn more. I have been a spiritual student for a long time, and I am a spiritual teacher. Did I mention how much I resisted this term "spiritual teacher?" My throat chakra just wouldn't let me be seen that way, let alone be recognized for it. Anyway,

I've come to learn that as students, we all eventually become our own teachers. We are all unique, and what works for one person may not work the same or as well for others.

To me, this applies to the chakras as well. I went online to see all the images for the chakras. There is some consistency, but the location, images, and names vary. If you think about it, in the Hindu tradition, for example, there was likely one person who meditated on their chakras and came up with some visuals, colors, sensations, emotions, and thoughts. After time, they decided that they knew where the exact locations were and decided to share this information with others. I'm sure some of these people had the same or similar experiences and others didn't. Yes, this book is partly about the chakras and most specifically the throat chakra. I only wish to claim to be an expert in my own experience of them, and I would like you to explore and become your own expert on the chakras.

A few weeks ago, I taught shamanism through the heart class, and part of what we did in the meditation was work on the back of the solar plexus. I always like to have the students share their experiences. One woman shared that she felt a strong connection with this chakra and that it was purple. Now, I don't think I could find anywhere that the solar plexus is purple. However, for her, it was purple, and I was elated that she had this experience. I don't know why her solar plexus is purple, but I'm glad it is and that she was the one who discovered it. I used to lead people in meditations, guiding them to experience the correct, corresponding colors as stated in various literature, and it never worked all that well, as it didn't work all that well for me. I feel much closer and connected to my chakras in my own unique experience, and I would love for you to do the same.

I studied and meditated on the chakras years ago, and I remember one author who explained it was best to go up and down the chakras like an elevator and then explode roses in front of the chakras, especially the heart center. The book I was following did not give a description of how to explode roses, so I would just imagine a large rose and let it explode into pieces in front of me. I don't remember ever benefiting from that part of the practice, but I was committed to growing spiritually and so did it long enough until I knew it wasn't meant for me. I don't have that book anymore and stopped doing those practices long, long ago because I outgrew them and moved onto other practices. My point is that many of the practices from the wide range of teachers or practitioners today may work well for you, but my heart's desire is to open a whole new door for you – a door that invites you to explore and work with your chakras as you and only you experience them. You are a unique being. There is nobody else in the world who has ever looked or been exactly like you. There is nobody the exact same today, and there never will be anyone who is precisely like you in the future. So why should your energy centers be the exact same as someone else's?

The most common way to access these energy centers is through the mind. We use our mind to focus on them and do all sorts of things. There is a great deal of music available that can help you get in touch with your chakras. I tried many of these, and none of them worked for me, but that doesn't mean they won't work for you. Please let me encourage you to pursue what attracts you. Maybe you would like to create your own music for the chakras. There are singing bowls for the chakras made of crystal or brass, and when played, in various ways, the vibration of the sound is felt and continues for a long time. The sounds are fantastic. I like singing bowls because the sound vibration they create fills the space and your being so beautifully, but they don't actually help me connect to my chakras near as much as meditation. I find focused meditation the best way to access and work with the chakras, and I would like you to try to join me in the exploration of the chakras.

Understanding Chakras with Heart/Emotion versus Mind

There are many diagrams and images in books and online that demonstrate the specific location of the chakras in the body. Some are accurate, and some are not so accurate. For years, when I worked with the chakras, I placed my attention in the front of my body, and I realized years later that sometimes I wasn't even totally in my body; I was doing the work as if the chakras were out in front. Once I realized this, I tried to place my attention in the middle of my body, and that helped me to be inside my body. I have come to realize that many of my students and clients do the same thing. For me, the actual chakras are mostly located along the inside of the spine, and when we work with them in front, we are only working at half strength. I discovered that the more I focus on the chakras at the spine, the more powerful the meditations, the more energy I feel, and therefore, the more powerful healing and empowerment I experience.

Chakra Locations

I would like to introduce the chakras here by simple location based on my experience and the experience of my students and clients when I do this exercise with them. If you are going to work with chakras, it is fundamental that you know the exact location in your own body, so you can focus your energy and breath there.

When working on a specific a chakra or chakras, I often ask my students if they would like me to touch their spine where the exact location is. This is usually helpful, so feel free to reach around with your hand and touch the location if you can. I remember working on the back of the solar plexus and placing an object with a soft, pointy part on it between the back of the solar plexus chakra and the chair. It was too hard to reach around and hold my finger there, so I found this extremely helpful. I'm a little embarrassed to say the object I used was a vacuum cleaner attachment, but it was the nearest thing to me at the time. I had been meditating and didn't want to stop for too long.

How to Locate Your Chakras

I am going to describe to you how I locate the chakras. There are an endless number of books out there on the chakras that have varying descriptions of chakra locations. I encourage you to go by feel, looking for either physical sensations, emotions, or both. Sometimes, the visual just comes, and that is totally fine too. Either at the beginning or end of one of your meditations, move your awareness up and down the spine, and then, starting with the root, see if you notice anything in the following locations as you practice the Full Rhythmic Breath. Remember to reach around and touch the locations physically if that helps. Take your time with this exercise and make it your own. You can repeat this, whether you experience something or not. I have provided a list of guidelines for easy location below:

- Root: bottom tip of coccyx

- Sacral: two to three inches below waist at back (inside spine)

- Solar plexus: feel in front first, soft spot below sternum where ribs come together; straight back from this location (inside spine)

- Heart: center of chest and back (inside spine)

- Throat: at the top of the hump on the spine (inside spine)

- Third eye: in center of forehead, back in the middle of head

- Crown: above center of head

While using the Full Rhythmic Breath, take some time to breathe into and out of each of these locations to become more familiar with them. There is no need to imagine colors, spinning, or images; this is simply to help you understand where the chakras actually are in your body. If colors or anything else comes for you, please just embrace it. Your centers are already communicating with you.

While meditating on my unique chakras as these locations, I decided to open myself to a more personal visual of my chakras to see if it varied from lotus petals or any other traditional representation. What I discovered was that my personal chakras are all represented by bouquets of flowers. Yes, they are not circular, with varying lotus petals or anything even close to that. When I open myself to experience my chakras as they are, in *my* being, along *my* spine, they are bouquets of flowers as follows:

1. Root Chakra: Red roses
2. Sacral Chakra: Daisies
3. Solar Plexus Chakra: Daffodils
4. Heart Chakra: Sun, with long and very bright rays
5. Throat Chakra: Irises with roots in Root Chakra and stem through Sacral, Solar Plexus, and Heart
6. Third Eye Chakra: Blue bells
7. Crown Chakra: Orchid plant

I was so grateful when I discovered this about the chakras because I always felt somehow challenged in creating or superimposing someone else's images on, or in, my chakras. This just felt so right because it was not from my mind; it was from my inner senses and knowing. Notice the seventh chakra is not a bouquet of flowers but an actual plant. I actually don't work there a whole lot. I find that when we work on the lower chakras, the crown automatically takes care of itself. It opens, it shines, and it does whatever it needs to do. It is ideal to work on the lower chakras for a long time before venturing into the crown chakra.

I used to be visual in my meditations, and now I mostly feel energy and emotions, as well as physical sensations. When I want a visual, it comes easy, but I find that I go deeper without the visual. In this practice, before I got the visual, I felt the energy of the chakra. I move my focus around the chakra, front to back and up and down, until I find the most intense location. They are there and just waiting for you to access them. Search to feel their energy. Each of your experiences of the chakras, if you explore with an open heart, will be slightly to largely different. I find it is much easier to access the chakras' energy and work with it when you have a more intimate connection with your own unique chakras.

Chakra by Location

Now that you have located your personal chakras, you want to get to know them better. You can read about them endlessly, and this is useful; I encourage you to take all that knowledge and bring it to your own experience, testing this knowledge to see if it is true.

I had a client on a one-week personal meditation retreat with me, and during our session together, she told me that the entire universe was in her solar plexus. This was a profound experience for her, and she described it to me as best she could, and of course, words could not explain. I had the same experience at different times, so I felt that I knew what she was talking about, but it still doesn't mean our experience was identical. She then said she felt kind of robbed. When I asked her why, she wanted to know why nobody ever told her that the entire universe was in her solar plexus. I couldn't help but smile. If someone told her the entire universe was in her solar plexus, even if she grew to believe it fully, it wouldn't give her the experience of knowing it at an experiential level.

My client will never forget how to experience this, but that also doesn't mean she can experience it at will. I gave her the meditation practices to do, and she did them; through these practices, she had this experience. This is what I am doing here. I am giving you some practices and encouraging you, as much as possible, to have your own experiences.

Throat Chakra and Supporting Chakras

This book is primarily about the throat chakra as it relates to your neck pain, and we will work intensely with the throat chakra in a further chapter. For now, we will continue to work with all the chakras because they are all connected. The throat chakra is not an isolated center; it is connected with one through seven. All the lower chakras below five (the throat charka) have an effect on it, and five has an effect on six and seven.

Across the board with my clients, I found that most of them have throat chakra issues, and as you'll remember, it can be one of the hardest chakras to heal. Part of the reason for that is that the energy runs up the spine and hits the bottleneck of the throat center. The energy naturally wants to come out as self-expression and, most importantly, expression of your purpose. Few of us feel grounded, stable, and safe enough in the root chakra to let our creative expression flow all the way up at the throat. Our creativity may be distorted or weak in the sacral chakra so that expression will be distorted or weak. The solar plexus chakra also wants to be expressed through the throat chakra, and we understand our own sense of power and truth; we understand how we may stifle our own power or sense of truth because that is how we've been conditioned.

Next, we get to the heart chakra, and we want to remember that all the lower three centers run through the heart before they get to the throat. If we have a small, broken, or sad heart because of all that happened to us in our earlier years and we don't process this, that darker energy comes up from the heart and into the throat, either getting stuck or expressing in ways we regret. That's why we often get a sense of hopelessness when the energy of the other chakras builds up in the throat, but there is hope! Let me help you get to know your chakras a little further so we can begin to work with them.

Chakra Meditation

Please get into the meditative posture and begin breathing fully. When it feels right, create a rhythmic breath by counting your heartbeats or pulse. Let this practice become comfortable and solid within you. When you are ready, feel into your confidence level, knowing where your chakras are located. You've done this practice before and have accomplished a sense of where they are located in your body. Let yourself feel the confidence of knowing you are ready to move on to a new practice.

Start with the root center. Breathe into its exact location as best you can. Tune into the energy of it

and any other details associated with it like images, colors, physical sensations, emotions, or even
smells. I want you to imagine that the root chakra
(and all the chakras) open front to back and notice
how that feels and if it feels right. You may want to
experiment with how this chakra operates for you
specifically. Take your time. I am going to work with
the notion that it opens front to back. I invite you to
breathe energy into the root chakra from the space
behind it. Inhale from the space behind it, and exhale
into the center, as if you are filling it up or lighting
it up or whatever wants to happen. Once you get
comfortable with this, see if you can inhale from the
front of the root chakra and exhale into it. Do this a
number of times until you have an experience of it.

Then I invite you to inhale from the space in front of
the chakra and the space behind the chakra at the
same time and exhale that energy into the chakra.
Notice how you imagine the energy coming in. Do
you see or feel the energy or both? We will work with
this further later on. Do this for about ten breaths,
and move onto the sacral chakra and do the same
thing, working all the way up to the third eye chakra.
Check in periodically throughout the meditation to
make sure you are breathing fully and that you feel
your heart beating, keeping it rhythmic. You also
want to check in occasionally with your spine and
posture, ensuring you are sitting straight.

Value of Journaling Meditations

If you're like me, you think you will remember everything that happened in the meditation, but you won't remember it a few days from now. Some of the details might even vanish in a few hours. It is good practice to write down all the details in your journal and read them before you do the practice again.

Years ago, I had a student who meditated every day. She was dedicated to her personal growth and the practices. She often wrote in her journal and loved the changes she was going through. Then, one day, she decided to read her meditation journal to review practices and the results she achieved. She could not believe what she discovered. For five months, she often got the guidance she needed to paint. She wrote in her journal and then forget about it. It took her five months of writing it down to realize how important this was to her. Once she realized it, she soon pulled out all her art supplies, expecting she would start painting and she didn't, couldn't, and wouldn't. She looked at her paints and her canvas every day and just couldn't do it. I asked if she had neck pain, as it seemed like a throat chakra issue. She did, and I gave her some practices to try. She started painting and even began using her art in her fashion design business, selling renderings to clients who didn't even exist before. Later in this book, you will learn how she moved to this success so you can too.

Please pat yourself on the heart for making it this far into this book. You have learned a great deal, and I would love to hear about your experience. Please also feel free to utilize my free guided meditations on my website.

I hope you gained a deeper understanding of the chakras and how they are connected. I encourage you to continue to explore your chakras on a personal level and trust you have made notes on your personal assessments in your journal. You can expect that as you change and grow, your chakras may change too and this often happens through energetic healing in the chakras. In the next chapter, we will move into healing the chakras and how and why to invite in spiritual support.

Chapter 8:

Introduction to Healing and the Chakras

"Healing is embracing what is most feared; healing is opening what has been closed, softening what has hardened into obstruction, healing is learning to trust life."
—Jeanne Achterberg

Hopefully, you have been practicing the meditations mentioned earlier, and if you're not, hopefully you will when the time is right for you. We will be taking this one step further in this chapter to touch into healing. I would first like to mention spiritual support, as it is a key component to deepening practices and getting the most out of them, although it is often overlooked in many spiritual paths.

What is spiritual support? Spiritual support is tuning into the invisible world and specifically invisible beings who we admire, adore, love, or feel a strong connection with or would even like to develop a strong connection with. Having spiritual support will help you on your journey to healing your throat chakra issues and can benefit you in any area of your life. These beings can be a deceased loved one like a grandmother or a deceased spiritual teacher or saint. The Angels, Buddha, and Jesus are popular beings to attune to, as they created great change in humanity and helped with our evolution. Spiritual support can come from ancient gods or goddesses like Shiva, Ganesh, Green Tara, Mohamed, Mother Mary, or any great being who we admire.

The benefits of our own spiritual development and healing can be tremendous through this practice. It's the great qualities that we recognize in them that exist in us. Through this kind of connection, we develop these qualities over time. We may be grateful for the unconditional love that a grandmother had for us, the power of Shiva, the joy of Ganesh, or how much change a spiritual master made in the world.

A spiritual being can be a living being as well like the Dali Lama or even Marianne Williamson. As I am the one providing these practices to you, you may want to tune into me and my spiritual energy to assist you in gaining the most from your meditations. This is not about the ego but an opening. We are all one, and the separation we experience is an illusion. Please join me in a meditation to call in the spirit of a great spiritual being.

Spiritual Support Meditation

When we begin our meditation, once we get into the posture and move into the full, rhythmic breath, we consciously call them in. It's as simple as placing the intention that you are asking and that they will respond. Notice how or where they show up. Do you get a visual, a physical sensation, emotion, or a sense of knowing? Maybe you can even feel their vibration. Notice where you sense them. Are they in front of you or behind you? Are they in front to strongly make themselves seen and known, or do they have your back and stand firmly behind you?

This may be difficult at first and I encourage you to trust this practice. Keep repeating this daily for a few minutes at the beginning of your meditation and as you meditate; it can help to tune into them periodically. This practice helps pull qualities and various sorts of power out of you that you do not recognize fully in yourself. Like attracts like, and the beings whom you are attracted to are specific to you. If you don't feel an attraction to any beings right now, you may want to Google spiritual being images. Close your eyes and meditate a few minutes with the intention that you will discover a being who you resonate with. Place your hand on your heart, and keep it there as you open your eyes. Scan the images in front of you slowly, noticing any sensations or emotions in your heart. You will likely be surprised at who shows up for you. Of course, you can always just simply meditate on this subject and ask your heart for guidance.

Once you have your being(s) and you call them in every day, you will notice your meditations improve. Don't we all do a better job when we feel deeply connected and strongly supported? This is a spiritual support that you just can't buy; it can only be created within you. All of the practices you do in this book will be better and more effective if you take a few minutes to do this daily.

Love

I talked about the power of breath and how it helps us heal. Now, I would like to talk about love. You know the saying, "Love heals all." This saying is true, but how do we make that work for us? If we haven't had a lot of love in our lives or haven't experienced deep love, this can be challenging. Even if we had loving relationships and easily experience love, we can never experience too much.

Just over twenty years ago, I led a group of friends in meditation on our usual Monday evening. I felt a great love within me and realized it was also outside of me and absolutely everywhere. I experienced love, and we breathed it in the air in that room. Love filled the entire Universe. It is one thing to think this intellectually, but to experience it is a whole different experience. I'm sure you have heard people say, "There is nothing but love; love is everything." Well, one way to help us tune into this all-pervading love is to repeat the word, and one of the best times to repeat it is during meditation.

Up until this point, you have been counting heartbeats with numbers. We are going to switch from counting with numbers to counting with the word "love" by creating a melody. We'll use eight counts in and eight counts out as an example. What I do is go up a musical scale for the first four and down a musical scale for the last four on the inhale and repeat the same on the exhale. This helps bring us more into our hearts and less into our mind because we no longer have to think as much by thinking of numbers. The word love becomes superimposed on and in our hearts and in our beings through the repetition. We can take this a step further and try to feel love every time we silently say the word. We say the word "love" silently, doing our best to feel the emotion of love.

This may take a bit of practice to get used to, and please do not expect perfect results right away with any of these practices. That's why we call them practices; we are practicing. Bringing in the spiritual support and the word "love" helps us not only prepare for our healing, growth, and empowerment but also begins to ease us into it.

Empower Your Heart Chakra

Let's take this a step further by empowering our hearts. So many of us today say, "Follow your heart" and somehow we think we know how to do that, or maybe we admit we don't entirely know what that looks or feels like. By empowering the heart, we can tune into it more and feel a deeper connection – a greater sense of who we are – and this makes it much easier to listen to the heart and follow it.

We are going to do an energizing practice that helps develop the heart chakra. In order to heal the throat chakra, we need to start developing and healing the other centers.

We will start with the heart because the throat chakra is the chakra that the heart is expressed most through. The clearer and stronger the heart center, the clearer and stronger the expression.

Heart Chakra Meditation

Let's begin by getting into the posture. Take your time to make sure your spine is straight and your head is lifted up toward the ceiling, feet flat on the floor and palms facing up. We can take a moment to notice what the regular breath is like before we take on the full breath. When it feels right, find your heartbeat, and begin to count heartbeats or seconds silently with the words love. Remember, it is like a musical scale going up for three or four counts and down for three or four counts. Once you are comfortable with this, we can move onto the next step. Please know it can take days or weeks to get comfortable with this way of counting.

After the inhale, the next step is to hold the breath physically in the lower abdomen and energetically in the heart center. To begin with, if your count is six, you will hold for six, and if it's eight, hold for eight, still counting with the word "love." Then exhale for the same count. This may feel uncomfortable or awkward at first, so please be patient with yourself. Know that the word "love" brings you unconditional love, which is very patient. Once you have mastered this, either today, tomorrow, or the next day, I encourage you to increase the hold portion to twice as much. If your count is eight, you are now holding for sixteen counts. The melody with the word "love" goes like this: up the scale "love, love, love, love," down the scale "love, love, love, love," up again "love, love, love, love," down, "love, love, love, love." This may feel very easy or very hard. The key to holding the breath for a double count is completing the exhale. Be sure to exhale all the air, and remember, you can always start over.

We are consciously bringing love into the heart and exhaling love. Remember, love is all-pervading; it is everywhere, within and without. You can imagine or feel yourself breathing in love, even breathing in all the love in the entire universe. If you don't feel or imagine much, we just fake it 'til we make it! This practice helps to energize and empower the heart center and will support us greatly in the work ahead.

Healing

Now is a good time to make use of these practices and begin to look at healing our wounds of the past. Why do we want to do this? Our physical pain is pretty much always associated with emotional or spiritual wounds or hurts of the past, which usually originated in our childhood. Therefore, we want to heal these wounds so that we can reduce the pain in our necks and shoulders. You are also reading this because you know your throat chakra could use some improvement. Maybe you feel stuck in your life or maybe you would like to express yourself in the world in a way that you are not doing right now.

Regardless of the pain we have or the desires and goals we long for, the fastest way to get there is through healing those old emotional wounds. It is far from fun and takes some courage, trust, and faith, and is so worthwhile. When I think of the value of healing, I think of the beautiful light and love that shines in your heart. It is meant to shine, and fundamentally, you are a being of light and love. The soul comes from light and love and will return to light and love. Becoming human creates a cover over that light and love. We are born into this earthly plane to our earthly parents in our earthly bodies, and we all get wounded in childhood. I have never met anybody who hasn't. Sure, some people may tell you, "My parents were so great. Sure, they may have made a few mistakes – nobody is perfect — but I had a wonderful childhood." However, they are wrong. These people are simply not ready to admit that they have any childhood wounds, let alone face them. We all have wounds of various degrees. Sometimes wounds go as far back as when we were invitro, and some wounds go back to infancy. Something happens, and we are emotionally or spiritually injured. The wound doesn't heal when there isn't anybody around who is able hold us in our pain and fear, and when there is nobody to love us through it unconditionally. We are not usually encouraged to cry the tears or to feel our emotions fully, so these emotions become stuck in us. The wound becomes familiar, and after a time, we don't even notice it.

You've heard the saying "Like attracts like." This saying applies to wounds as well as people. The wound attracts more of the same, and this repeats throughout our lives. We end up with patterns that we usually don't recognize at all, or when we do, it is a well-ingrained pattern, a pathway for the same type of wound repeated over and over. This remains in our subconscious until we find a means to let the wound come to the surface, to let it become conscious.

Is it beginning to make sense as to why you may feel stuck in some area(s) of your life? This is why we do our best in meditation to access the subconscious through the full breath so that we can feel the trapped emotions and the pain of the distant past and give ourselves the gift of feeling all of it in the here and now so that it no longer holds us back; it can no longer cover our light in the same way. When we do this long enough, our behavior begins to change. We are not using the mind to change the behavior. There is so much out there on how to control the mind to create change, but this can only go so far.

Using the mind doesn't get to the root of the problem. Going as deeply as we can into the chakras, the energy centers that hold all of who and what we are, allows us to heal the problem and the result is that our behavior changes; what we say changes. The triggers that used to prompt reactions no longer exist. We change for the better in permanent ways, and the soul is so satisfied because that is part of its mission. The soul signs up for the wounds that hurt us so that the soul can heal and evolve in this human body. The soul will go on forever, and this life here is but one small stage of its evolution. Let's work together here and now and do what we can to access the wounds of the past and remove the covers that hide your light so that you can begin to shine more and more every day.

One of my clients – I'll call him John – who initially came to me with neck pain and excruciating hip pain insisted that he had those wonderful, loving parents and had a great childhood. Everyone around him was kind and loving. He admitted to a few childhood wounds that he suffered but dealt with years ago. One day, he called me up in desperation that his hip suddenly hurt so badly he could hardly walk. I did an online healing session, and he went back to the little boy in the boy's restroom who was threatened sexually by a bully at school. I helped him feel into the fear and terror that younger boy felt and helped him move through it. It was a memory he hadn't thought about in decades, and when he first remembered it in the session, he felt no emotion. Once the emotion came, I helped him move through it, pulling the toxic energy out of his sacral chakra. Once the session finished, he could walk again, and by the next morning, he was completely pain free. He later began to uncover terrible abuse by his grandmother, and this man, who went to the chiropractor one to four times a month for over forty years because of neck and back pain, has been pain-free for months. Not only is his pain gone, but his heart is also shining in a way it never did. He experiences a level of joy and happiness he could only imagine previously. As you can see, healing wounds is extremely worthwhile.

Do you want what John now has? You can have that. You can uncover that beautiful heart of yours that wants to shine the light and love that is inherent in you. You made the com-

99

mitment to yourself earlier on, and now would be a good time to review that. You've practiced the meditations, which essentially puts that commitment into action. These basic meditations can be healing in and of themselves. If you felt any uncomfortable emotions during any of the meditations, please do not stop meditating when they arise. The breath may change and go from smooth to jagged, or it may become more difficult to breathe. Please continue breathing in the best way you can, breathing through the emotion or physical discomfort. I promise you will come out of the other side. It may return again and again, but your entire being wants to feel all these repressed emotions until they are complete, so you can more freely move into uplifting emotions like joy and happiness. Feeling these emotions and moving through them uncovers the light and love of the heart. It removes the darkness so your light can shine.

Locating and Healing Wounds

Let's move into locating our wounds. I first learned to locate wounds in a therapy session with an amazing therapist who practiced Hakomi, body-centered psychotherapy, developed by Ron Kurtz. When my therapist helped me discover my wound, it was so big that it was larger than my body and was out in front of me, attached to my heart chakra and solar plexus. I was ready and willing to do whatever it took to make some serious changes in my life. My therapist helped me move through that painful experience, and then invited me to a weekend workshop for lay counselors who she taught in a community program. She told me that she was impressed with how open I was to heal and admired the difficult work I was so willing to do. I initially felt a little out of place, but once I settled into it, I discovered it was the perfect place for me. Everyone wanted to heal and most of them wanted to help heal others. That was about twenty-three years ago. I brought the Hakomi work into my meditations, uncovering and healing emotional wound after emotional wound. I later studied Hakomi again when I earned a diploma in Jin Shin Do acupressure, using Hakomi to help my acupressure clients heal their wounds. I remember finding multiple emotional wounds in my neck and when working with others, finding the same in them. I also discovered Peter Levine's work, somatic experiencing and somatic touch, and discovered and healed wounds through those methods. While practicing shamanism, I discovered methods to locate and heal others' emotional and spiritual wounds as well as my own. Meditation has served me greatly in healing wounds. Like I said earlier, the Full Rhythmic Breath is the technique that the others didn't have. The hara breathing came pretty close in acupressure. I now practice Hurqalya Healing, a form of energy healing developed by Puran and Susanna Bair, and I bring into that aspects of other healing work I have done and work with wounds located in the physical body, energetic body, and specifically the chakras.

Recently, I had a spiritual teacher tell me that I healed all my wounds, but when I began writing this book, issues still came up. I knew one day I would write a book, but like most people who want to write a book, all sorts of things get in the way, but mostly it's ourselves that get in the way. Whatever stopped me from writing a book earlier came up, and I was

101

able to quickly and easily heal that and move forward. I will tell you that emotional and spiritual wound healing usually becomes more difficult once you start, but the more success you have, the easier and faster it gets until you find your level of happiness, peace, joy, and contentment increases and replaces the negative self-talk, sadness, despair, etc. Happiness becomes the daily norm.

All these methods help one locate emotional wounds by locating them as physical sensations in the body. If you feel an emotional wound as well, all the better. We can work with the physical, emotional, and mental wounds. If you already have physical pain, the first thing to do is breathe into that pain wherever it is located in the body. Then try and find the emotion, though the emotion can come first too. Say you keep noticing a particular emotion coming up and it won't go away. Let's say you feel sadness around some news you received from a friend; you have been thinking about the news a lot, and you feel sad. You can meditate on the emotion and then find the location of the emotion in the body. Often, the more intense or long-lasting emotions in your current life are rooted back to wounds in your childhood, which I will discuss more later. Let me help you locate a wound or two.

Chakra Healing Meditation

Please sit in the posture, back straight and feel flat on the floor. Lift the crown up toward the ceiling and bring your awareness to your spine, following it up and down. This can help us get into our bodies. Take on the full breath, breathing into the lower abdomen and make it rhythmic, silently using the word "love" to count the heartbeats. Invite in your spiritual support and once you feel this support, focus on breathing in their love into your heart every time you say the word "love" silently. Do this for a few minutes. Notice your level of safety. It's important that we feel safe before doing this kind of exercise. Make any necessary adjustments. Spend some time, at least five minutes, breathing love into and out of your heart center. Breathing love allows the heart center to become energized and rejuvenated. Feel free to just continue with this practice if you want and continue on to the remainder next time.

Breathing fully, counting heartbeats with the word love, let a memory come of any difficult moment or time in your life. Let the memory come to you. Notice the first one that comes; let yourself remember what it was like and how it felt. Keep breathing fully. Notice if you feel any sensation(s) in your body. Take a moment, while staying with the memory, to scan your body for any physical sensations. If you notice something, that is great! Keep your focus on the physical sensation while you still hold onto the memory. If you didn't feel anything in the body, do a slower scan, starting with the top of your head and moving downward, very slowly scanning your body, looking for any physical sensation. Notice whatever shows up. If more than one location shows up, go with the prominent one.

Now we are going to send energy from the heart to the location. Exhale your heart's energy from the heart center to the physical sensation for your count, still using the word "love." Then inhale the energy from the location back to your heart. Continue to breathe fully and count the heartbeats with the word "love" on the melody. You can put the intention of sending all the love and light in your heart center to the area, which we will now refer to as the wound. Then inhale the energy of the wound into your heart center. It may seem kind of scary to inhale the wound's energy into the heart, but the heart is so powerful; it can easily integrate it. Notice if there is an emotion that arises with the physical sensation. Continue to do the breath, regardless of the emotion. Let yourself feel the emotion fully. If tears start to flow, let them flow, and just do your best to continue with the practice. You can just take it one breath at a time. If you only feel the physical sensation, that is great too. Continue with this practice until the physical and/or emotional symptoms are completely gone. Your beautiful light and love-filled heart has integrated the wound.

You have done an excellent job of locating wounds and healing them. Please continue to practice this meditation every day for at least one week. It is a practice you will have for the rest of your life, and you will hopefully return to it again and again.

You have learned to call in spiritual support, and this is worth doing every time you meditate and at any other time in the day. You have learned how to heal through meditation, how to locate wounds, experience the emotions and let them move through you, transforming themselves. You have not only physically located your chakras, but you have learned more about your own chakras and what they represent to you. We will continue on this healing journey in the next chapter, going deeper into the chakras and deeper into healing.

Chapter 9:

Going Deeper with Meditation and Chakra Energy Work

"The wound is the place where the Light enters you."

—Rumi

In healing neck pain and the throat chakra, I found that creating safety is so helpful. Yes, you created safety in your meditation space. It feels good, and you feel safe in doing the practices. To move on to further work and to create space for healing and empowerment, I would like to help you create a deeper sense of safety.

You can begin by pulling out your journal. Please write about how safe you felt in the world as a child. How safe did it feel to express your emotions, dreams, wants, and beliefs? What level of safety did you experience at the various stages of growing up? Give yourself a rating on a scale of one to ten for the safety level you experienced as you grew up and in your adult life through career, relationships, parenthood, travelling, health, religion, spirituality, etc. What is your capacity for taking risks? How did you assess whether something was safe? What were your hidden beliefs or conscious beliefs around safety? How safe in the world do you feel today? Who or what has helped you with your level of safety and who or what has reduced it? Please provide all the time you need for this exercise. This exercise will provide you with a personal assessment of your previous and current level of safety in your life.

There is a certain level of safety associated with all the chakras that affects how the throat chakra expresses itself or holds that expression in. How can you easily and comfortably express your truth if you have an underlying sense of fear and a conscious or subconscious lack of safety? If it's too scary to say what you mean, ask for what you want, or say how you honestly feel, it's next to impossible to be authentic. All our authenticity remains inside, and we have a hard time recognizing it or don't know what is real or not. Our overall level of safety originates in the root center. People often talk about feeling grounded or ungrounded and being in their head or out of their body. A strong and stable root center creates a certain amount of safety and prevents us from easily being knocked over. With a strong and vibrant root center, we know that there's not a lot that could happen to us that we can't get through. Even when terrible things happen, we know that, as hard as it may be, we will make it through. When the root center is wounded, lacks energy, or even has too much to make it healthy, we don't make decisions that are in our best interest. This applies to all areas of life – health, relationships, career, spirituality, creativity, or even rest and relaxation.

We are going to start by working with the root chakra, and then we will move onto the other chakras.

Let's meditate. This time, please have your journal with you and open to the page where you just wrote about your level of safety throughout life. Please review that and keep it close by, as you may want to open your eyes occasionally and use it in this meditation.

Bringing in Love Meditation

Take your time to make sure you are in the perfect posture. Feel your feet on the floor and your seat in the chair, shoulders back and relaxed. Begin breathing in the Full Rhythmic Breath until it feels natural, and call in your spiritual support. Give yourself as much time as you need to get in tune with who is with you and the support they offer.

Let's locate the root center at the base of the coccyx or wherever you feel your exact location is. Breathe into the root center from the back, inhaling the energy from the space behind you and into the center for five to ten breaths. Then inhale from the space in front of you and into the root for five to ten breaths. Continue to breathe fully; inhale from the front and back of the center, and exhale into the center. Continuing to breathe fully, see if you can inhale love into this center as you breathe. Love is everywhere; it is all-pervading.

If you don't feel it, that's fine; take the time to imagine the love you feel for a loved one and let yourself feel that in your heart. Once you have that feeling, breathe that into the root center from front and back. You can use the word "love" instead of numbers to count the heartbeats and this helps feel the love even more. Feel yourself filling the root chakra up with love. It may even become bigger or brighter. Notice your experience as you fill the root chakra up with love. Now, let yourself feel you are holding your root chakra with love. You can let go of the inhale from front and back and just breathe into and out of the root chakra filled with love. As you are holding your root chakra with love or remaining attuned to the love in the root, think of the level of safety in the world that you experienced at an earlier time. Let the memory come to you, whatever comes up first. Let yourself feel whatever emotions come and even look for them – fear, anger, whatever comes. Imagine they are in the root center.

Once you feel that fully, allow yourself to breathe into it fully so you feel the discomfort completely. This is not easy, but it is temporary, and you will get through it. Continue to breathe love into and out of the chakra, along with the memory and any emotions or even thoughts associated with it. You know you have healed it when the emotion changes.

This will happen naturally, and then one of three things will happen. First, the emotion will change into another much more comfortable emotion like peace or love, and you definitely know healing has happened at a deep level. Secondly, another difficult emotion will arise, and you will breathe through the new emotion in the same way. Lastly, a new memory may arise, and you can start again breathing into it with love and holding yourself like a loving mother holds her child in pain. When you feel like you have completed all your healing work for that sitting, I invite you to breathe into the root center with love, acknowledging any subconscious wounds that did not show up today.

On the exhale, imagine any remaining memories that cannot come to the surface down and into the earth. You exhale this with the intention you are exhaling the energy of the subconscious wounds remaining in the root center, especially the ones specific to safety. Do this for five to ten breaths. You can also set the intention that you are exhaling all that is held in the root that no longer serves you around safety, or whatever intention that feels ideal for you.

Exhale it as deeply as you can, even all the way down to the center of the earth. Know that our mother earth has all the capacity to process and integrate it. When it feels right, inhale the unconditional love from mother earth up into the root center and let

it fill it up like the love you inhaled earlier. Do this
complete exercise as long as it feels appropriate.

Do this exercise once or twice a day until your internal
sense of safety has increased to a level that you are happy with.

Resistance to Meditating Daily

Remember in the beginning of the book when I first started
meditating? It took me eight entire months of sitting before I felt anything at all, and whatever it was that I felt was
incredibly brief. I still kept going. I kept meditating every
day, and I started to feel better and better. I noticed that if
I didn't meditate, I didn't feel as good. Remember, I didn't
start meditating out of curiosity or to become spiritual. My
reason was strong – my deceased brother advised me to do
it, and I discovered that he said this to help me get out of
the depression. And it worked. I knew I had to do it every
day. I got off the medication and never had to go back on.
It also helps to have a teacher. I had teachers in physical
form as well as through books. If you want to play a musical
instrument like a musician you admire, you first need to
learn to play, and you can do that on your own or you can
get a teacher. However, what needs to follow is you have to
practice consistently, and this is where most people give up.
Whenever we take on something new that is important to
us, our stuff is going to come up and try to prevent us from
practicing. Everything that prevented you from even trying
to be a musician in the past will surface, and most of the

time, you won't even notice it. Over time, you will no longer want to practice.

The first thing to help you continue is to remember the reason you are doing it. If you just don't feel like meditating, best thing to do to combat any kind of resistance is to sit and feel your resistance and any other emotions that go along with it. Feel whatever it is that prevents you from doing something – the fear, the sadness, the unworthiness, the feelings that you are not good enough, etc. Susan Jeffers wrote *Feel the Fear and Do It Anyway*, and that book helped me learn that no matter what I try to do, fear is inevitable. It's normal, so just feel it.

When I sold my house, my interior design business, and all my belongings except two suitcases, which I put into storage, I was going to move to Costa Rica and start a new life. In this new life, I would walk slowly, as I had always gone so fast before. The truth was I was in the depths of the dark night of the soul. I had mastered my business in interior design and kept trying to master it in different ways. I would expand my business or develop a new aspect of it until I mastered that and then looked for something else in it to master, completely unaware of what I was doing. As soon as I would start to slip into the dark night of the soul, I would find a new way to experience success until nothing fulfilled me anymore and there was no more looking. If you are not sure what the dark night of the soul is, I think Hazrat Inayat Khan sums it up perfectly:

"There can be no rebirth without a dark night of the soul, a total annihilation of all that you believed in and thought that you were."

The dark night of the soul to the Sufi's is a stage of "un-learning." One goes from mastering or being an expert at something – which is most often in career but can also be experienced in parenthood, marriage, health, or spirituality – and then goes into the dark night of the soul where nothing satisfies us anymore. It can come on suddenly or gradually, and one's preconceived notions about everything begins to change into not knowing.

I remember well at Christmas a few years ago I asked my older brother how he was doing. He said he didn't know. I asked him how he felt, and he said, "I don't know how I feel." I then asked what he did know, and he said he really didn't know anything. The expression on his face was of one who felt lost. Now, my brother had achieved outstanding success in his field, worked way too many hours, and it was just months after that that he quit his job.

People really suffer in the dark night of the soul, and nobody gets through it easily. I believe I was in the dark night for almost a decade. One almost always needs to find a spiritual teacher to help them through to the next step of unity consciousness, which is a stage of complete contrast to the dark night. Life becomes incredibly bright, and one feels connected to and a part of everything and everyone.

When I found IAM Heart, I was in the dark night and would have peak experiences of unity consciousness but didn't know how to stay there. I kept falling back into the dark night. Fairly early into IAMU, I moved more deeply into unity consciousness and within months was able to stay there. My entire world changed. Everything was so vibrant and alive, my senses were heightened, and I felt ongoing joy to be alive.

When I wanted to, I could look at anything and feel it as a part of me and me, a part of it. I was in love with the world and everything in it. At times, I would almost feel manic, but never experienced the opposite depression.

Most people I work with are in this transition, moving from the dark night to unity consciousness. It is the most difficult transition in life to make but the most worthwhile. I know many people who get to this stage and, decades later, die in this stage. Most people never get to this stage, so not everyone goes through it, but the ones who do, in my opinion, are beginning to get in touch with their true calling, their soul's purpose.

How is this related to the throat chakra? The throat chakra is where the "expression" of your truth and your soul's purpose gets stuck energetically. Wounds of the past get in the way of your natural expression of truth, who you are in the world, and what you are here to do and be. This is the underlying reason for this book and why I want to help you heal your throat chakra issues so that it can shine the way it was meant to.

Back to my story of leaving everything behind. I'm sure you can imagine leaving your home and everything and everyone you loved. My heart guided me strongly, and even then, I listened to and followed my heart. At that time, I lived in a beautiful float home at Fisherman's Wharf in downtown Victoria, B.C. Canada. To everyone around me, I had the perfect life – a beautiful home, a successful business, two great grown children, and lots of friends, and I hiked, kayaked, traveled, and attended many spiritual workshops and events. Why would I want to leave?

Well, nothing satisfied me anymore. My work, which used to be so fulfilling, didn't fulfill me anymore, regardless of what I tried. Anyway, that's a whole different story and a stage of spiritual development that is inevitable for most spiritual seekers. My point is that I welled up with fear when I sorted everything I owned to sell or give away. I thought, "What am I doing? I don't even speak Spanish!" I stopped, sat down, and breathed into the fear and let myself feel it all. I continued to feel all my fear until it dissipated, and then the emotion of fear changed into happiness and joy. I felt how my heart guided me on this adventure, and that is how I kept going.

I ended up not living in Costa Rica and instead traveled for twenty months, becoming a backpacker for the first time at age forty-seven and traveling to every country in South America, five countries in Africa, and was in and out of Costa Rica and Panama multiple times. I've been told a number of times I should write a book on my travels, but this book is what is in my heart. I can't tell you how many times I felt fear when I traveled in these developing countries, and every time, I just breathed into it. I think it saved my life more than once. Thank you, Susan Jeffers, for one of my favorite mottos – feel the fear and do it anyway.

Where would you like to apply this practice in your life? Let's apply it to the practice of sitting inside your heart. My strong intention for you in this practice is to help you move through some fear so that you can loosen up and even break away some of what is stuck in your throat chakra and what may be holding you back. I want your heart and throat chakras to shine. Let's explore this in meditation.

Sitting Inside Your Heart Meditation

Sit very straight in the posture in your safe meditation space and take on the full breath. Practice the full breath until it feels natural. Make sure to exhale completely, squeezing the abdominal muscles to expel all the air. When it feels right, find your heartbeat and make your breath rhythmic. Do this until it feels very comfortable and natural. Take as much time as you need to invite your spiritual support. I invite you to breathe in love – breathe in the love that is all-pervading, the love that fills the entire Universe. Breathe it from all around you and into your heart center. Exhale all that love into your heart, filling it up like a vessel. Once this becomes comfortable, after the inhale, hold the breath physically in the lower abdomen and energetically in the heart center. Exhale this love into the heart center, filling it up.

Once this feels comfortable, bring light into the breath. Inhale light and love into the heart center, hold it there and exhale it into the heart center. You can imagine your pericardium that encases your heart – the protective covering. Imagine that you are stretching the pericardium with the love and light that is in your heart on the exhale. Make sure to keep your long, rhythmic breath. Let it stretch and expand a little more on every exhale, replenishing the love and light on every inhale. Notice how it feels to expand your heart center in this way. Keep expanding the energetic pericardium on every exhale until it reaches out to your shoulders and then beyond, every breath making it larger and larger. Give yourself the time and space to keep going with this exercise until the energetic pericardium is stretched well beyond belief and the heart center extends well beyond your physical form.

Once you feel yourself sitting inside your heart center, keep the breath inside your enormous heart. Feel your giant heart breathing. Continue to inhale and exhale love and light. Experience yourself as the light and love that is your heart. You are your heart.

Know that every time you do this practice, you grow and heal, so one cannot do this too often. This is a practice I even do sometimes when I am out in the world. When I talk with friends or even a stranger, sometimes I remember to just be my heart, and I let it expand, becoming bigger than me. It always helps me feel a stronger connection to the person or people I am with; this way, I definitely listen more thoroughly, take so much more than words, and what comes out of my mouth is authentic. To me, this practice is well worth the effort.

Power of the Heart Chakra

I love to be in touch with my heart and use it often in making decisions. I had been on my spiritual journey for about five years when a friend tried to teach me muscle testing. She worked with me, and none of the methods she presented seemed to work well for me. Maybe they were working, but I couldn't help but feel doubt. While she taught me the method where you stand still and ask yourself a question to see if your body moves forward or back, indicating a yes or no answer, I started to focus on my heart. When I did that, I automatically knew the answer and there was no doubt. She was delighted, and so was I.

At the time, I changed my diet and started to use this method in the grocery store. I would hold up certain foods to my heart and close my eyes for a brief second, or even place my left hand on the food and breathe the energy of the food into my heart. It is a no-fail practice to me. Twenty years later, I still use that practice and use it widely. You can use it when thinking of buying absolutely anything. Using this method to determine whether or not I should take certain supplements has been a saving grace. I believe that meditating on the heart helps us follow it and live with much less self-doubt.

The heart center is the most powerful center of all the chakras. When we develop this chakra and make it strong and bright, we can use it to heal all the other chakras. We can send its energy to each of the chakras just like we sent the energy to the physical sensations we felt in our bodies earlier. There are numerous meditations we can do to heal any chakra with the heart chakra's powerful energy. This book is not big enough to include them all, and I encourage you to experiment on your own or sign up for one of my courses.

While the heart center is the most powerful center and it is ideal to keep doing practices to heal and empower that center, we can also do a number of practices to heal and empower all the centers. When I first started working with the chakras over twenty years ago, it was strictly working with the mind, using my imagination. I find that working with the breath and energy and accessing emotions and/or memories creates the best results. It's not just about having an interesting experience; it's about changing to become who you truly are.

We practiced breathing love into the centers while silently saying the word "love," and we practiced breathing love and light into the heart center. Taking these practices to another level, you can try inhaling love and light into each of the centers, one at a time, and holding it in there and then exhaling that light and love. I encourage you to start with inhaling in the back first for some breaths, then the front, and then both, focusing on the exact location of the particular chakra you work with. I like to start with the root and work my way up, staying longer at whichever chakra feel likes it needs the most work. It is natural for uncomfortable emotions or physical sensation to come up. This is just a wound that wants to be healed. Whether you know what it is related to or not doesn't matter. It is simply a part of you that wants to heal.

Please stay on that chakra, if and when this happens, and keep breathing. Let the breath, light, and love heal the wound. When I work with love and light, I like to work with the words "love and light." I say, "love" on one heartbeat and then "and light" on the second heartbeat, "love" on the third and "and light," on the fourth, going up the musical scale, followed by "love" on the throat, "and light" on the sixth, "love" on the seventh and "and light," on the eighth. It helps me feel the love and light more and helps to keep me focused on the practice. I do this practice every morning at the beginning of my meditation, breathing into each chakra about five times. Of course, if and when something comes up, I stay wherever I am until it has passed and the chakra is filled with light and love. I find this starts my meditation and my day so beautifully, as it is healing and empowering. Doing this is like a quick little workout that you couldn't pay me to miss. If you do this practice before bed, notice that it helps with sleep or dreams.

Of course, you are reading this with neck pain, and I encourage you to spend lots of time on the throat chakra with this practice. Breathe into the pain, breathe into the stiffness. Feel how big each of the chakras are. You are healing and cleansing the chakras. We brush our teeth every day – morning and night – so why wouldn't we do the same with the chakras? The chakras become dirty, just like the teeth do. Over time, since all the lower chakras support the ones above them, you will become aware of which chakras supporting the throat chakra need work. Any and all work that we do on the lower chakras helps the work in the throat chakra hold.

Are you still calling in spiritual support? I find that once you get into the habit, it only takes seconds to call in support, and it helps more and more over time with these practices. I find it especially useful to call in a spiritual teacher. As you are learning these practices from me and doing the practices, calling me in will improve the practices for you. Remember, we are all one. You already know how to do all these practices; it is just a matter of accessing them. By imagining me there with you, you will feel my support and, therefore, feel the practices more intensely.

This has been a full chapter. You have taken yourself to a deeper level of safety, learned practices to further develop your heart center, and to "feel the fear and do it anyway." You've learned a bit about the dark night of the soul and how this relates to the throat chakra and stuck energy. You have learned to practice sitting inside your expanded heart center and how to use love and light to heal wounds energetically held in your chakras. I bow to you for coming this far, for being so brave and creating the change you so desire. You deserve to have your throat chakra shine, and all of this work is serving you toward that goal.

In the next chapter, we will explore light and how to access and further develop the light that is inherently a part of us.

Chapter 10:

Light Beings

"When you possess light within, you see it externally."
—Anais Nin

You are a Light Being; I am a Light Being. We are all Light Beings! To me, this is such an exciting chapter. How many of us know we are Light Beings? Now, this chapter may possibly be too far out there for you, and I am willing to take the risk to include it here because it is my truth and I would love more than anything to help you find your light. Whether or not you had an experience similar to mine doesn't matter. You are a Being of Light, and I can help you access this truth. This experience came to me firsthand when Light Beings from I don't know where began visiting me, and I'll never forget how it began.

I moved to Vancouver, Canada from Vancouver Island to fulfill my childhood dream of becoming a fashion designer. At the age of fifty-two, I moved from a beautiful house to a tiny apartment right on English Bay close to downtown Vancouver to get a diploma in fashion design. One day, while sweeping the floor, my grandma's spirit showed up. It was incredible. I never had that kind of experience before, so I kind of doubted she was there or that it was actually happening, so I went back to sweeping. I tried to ignore her, thinking I was making it up. My grandma and I were so close through my teens right up until she died while I was traveling in Africa. She was one of my best friends ever and my friends loved her too.

Anyway, finally, she said to me, "Cheryl, please sit down. Please sit down."

"Woah!" I thought, sitting down. I don't remember the conversation anymore, but I remember that she said all kinds of encouraging things to me and told me how she saw me. It made me cry because I could feel my grandmother's deep love and care for me. While I felt some of the truth in her words, the experience was somewhat overwhelming. That was when the Light Beings showed up. I wasn't even meditating. I was just sitting there, overwhelmed by my grandma, and the room became filled with these very tall rods of golden light. "Have I gone crazy?" I wondered.

Well, the Light Beings stayed and moved around. The room was so bright with them. My grandma asked me to meditate, and I sat there and breathed in all her love and the light from these Light Beings in the room. After that, they started coming to me in almost every meditation. One or a few would stand behind me, and they would stretch my neck up, sometimes so much that it hurt. It all seemed so strange at first, but I grew to enjoy the experiences, which were quite intense. I loved how the room would become brighter, and I could feel light within me. Later, it was like one of the Light Beings would enter my body, and I would become one of them. Oh, those were the days. This went on for several months.

So, why were the Light Beings there, and what were they doing? Why did they stretch my neck? Now, I understand what I couldn't understand then. The Light Beings wanted me to shine my light, and it was stuck in my throat chakra. They stretched or activated my throat chakra. I wasn't letting the truth of who I was shine, and God and the Light Beings wanted to see me shine. In the same way, I want to see you shine. Your light is meant to shine.

It was early in the time of Light Beings when I started teaching my fellow classmates in the design program. The problem was that when I would teach, the Light Beings would come and stretch some of my students' necks. A number of them also noticed that the room would get brighter. Now, these were all beginner meditators! They shared their experiences and asked why this happened, and I didn't know what to say. I was scared that if I told my students there were Light Beings in the room stretching their necks, they wouldn't come back. I started to ask the Light Beings to keep it down and leave my students alone. They did draw back on their participation in my classes but not entirely. Eventually, I told one of the students who became a good friend. Her neck was stretched the most. She loved it and started to see Light Beings occasionally in her apartment. It took a long time for me to share this with any of the teachers in IAMU, and none of them had an explanation for it. I did eventually meet someone else who experienced the same kind of Light Beings; they were as blown away by the experience as I was.

Do you need to experience Light Beings the way I did? Probably not; however, part of the source of your neck pain is likely a subconscious fear of allowing your light to shine brightly. Every one of us is a beautiful and unique soul who was born into a human body, and we are meant to shine. I used to have people tell me I had a lot of light, but I couldn't experience it. It took me years to experience my own light, and it was through healing my chakras that I was able to get more in touch with it and let it shine. This journey was not easy for me, and I was a slow study.

My husband saw the light in me the first time we met. I'll never forget when he first told me. At a retreat, he stood with a group of people and looked over at me. We had never been introduced or spoken to each other. I sat with a friend at a table, and my future husband walked up to me, sat down, and introduced himself. Next, he asked me if I knew how much light I had. I admired this man when I first met him, and he was one of teachers. In response, I said no, I didn't, and he seemed surprised. Then, he asked if I experienced a lot of light in my meditations. That I could answer yes to, as the Light Beings had been around for a long time.

We can see the light in others in their eyes. Do you notice how some people's eyes just sparkle? Oh, how I love sparkly eyes. However, whether or not others can see light in our eyes, we all have a lot of light. We have so much light – every one of us – because we are Light Beings. Whether you believe this to be true or not, please humor me and work with me on this. You can even start with the affirmation "I am a Light

Being" or "I am a Being of Light." The more we realize this, the more we heal our wounds that cover the light; it's like we start to pull the light from inside us, loosening up the dark wounds that cover it. You are one of those people who is meant to walk into a room and light it up.

In the last chapter, I introduced bringing in love and light. Just saying these words benefits us. Using these words to count heartbeats, in the melody that we created, helps us in so many ways.

How much light do you have in your eyes? I certainly did not see any light in my eyes, not that I ever tried, but some others did. I was given a practice some years ago by one of the deceased spiritual masters who I called in for spiritual support. I received a small picture of him as a gift. I loved the picture, and it meant a lot to me. I would like to share this practice with you because it helped me get in touch with my light and let it shine. You can do this practice with a picture or imagine some great spiritual being sitting across from you. You could also try imagining me sitting across from you simply because this practice was given to me and I do it a lot.

Light Meditation

Begin with the meditative posture and Full Rhythmic Breath, using the word "love," "light," or "love and light" to count heartbeats. Open your eyes for a few seconds and look into the person's eyes in the picture. If you use a great being of whom you do not have a physical image, just do the exercise with eyes closed and use your imagination to follow along. I will lead the practice from the point of having the picture in front of you.

Look into their eyes with your eyes open and then close your eyes and try to remember their eyes. All this time, we are energetically focusing the breath in the heart center however that is easiest and most comfortable for you. Keep the belly moving well. Continue to open your eyes and look into the eyes of this great being and close your eyes until you remember the eyes and the face well in your mind.

Then, imagine that this being is exhaling his/her heart's energy and white light from their heart up to their eyes, into your eyes, and down to your heart. Please feel free to read this sentence over. The shape is like three sides of a rectangle – they exhale up to their eyes, across to your eyes and down into your heart. While they are exhaling, you are going to inhale this white light from their heart, through their eyes, into your eyes, and down into your heart. On your exhale, you will send this light and heart energy from your heart, back to theirs through the same channel – the eyes. You can absolutely bring love into this practice. Feel free to open your eyes at any time briefly to look at the picture of the being in front of you again.

I find this to be a pretty advanced practice and this may take some time to get used to, but again, it is so worthwhile. Feel the heart connection between the two of you grow. Feel how this being wants to see your light shine in the world as it is meant to. Let him/ her bring out the greatness in you. Let him/her bring out all the light that is hidden in your heart. Let his/ her love for you fill your heart. Let yourself feel how it is clearing the throat chakra. The light and love move from heart chakra, through the throat and up to the third eye chakra. When it comes back on the inhale, it again passes through the throat chakra. The heart center is known most strongly for love and the sixth center known most strongly for light.

You can take this practice to a more advanced level if you so wish. Once you have done this practice for at least a week, or even longer, you can take it to a more powerful level. After you inhale the light from the great being's heart and eyes into your heart, hold your breath and hold the energy there for as long as is comfortable. Feel the light and love filling up your heart. Feel the light and love fill up your entire being. Over time, you may even feel it fill up your heart center until your heart center is larger than you.

We experienced love and light when we learned to sit inside our expanded heart center, and now, we can experience light and love and connect and commune with a great spiritual master.

To work further with light, please keep exploring your own chakras in meditation. I have given you some practices, and while doing them, I encourage you to discover exactly where in the body you access the light in each chakra. Is it way in the front, the back, top, or bottom of your body? Do you access it more if you extend the breath for a further two counts? What happens if you meditate longer? Do you give yourself time to get over that hump of wanting to stop? How do you feel when you access your own inner light?

I know I can't help but to smile big. You deserve to access your light, and you deserve to let it shine. Think of Jesus and his halo; his parents were shown with halos too. How many images can you find online with light radiating from the heart, from heaven, or even from the hands? We are Light Beings, and we are meant to shine. The practices I provided are but a few that you can use to access your light and become the radiant being that you are. By accessing your light, it helps to heal your neck issues and brings your throat chakra in tune with your entire energetic system. If you want to make a difference in the world, let your light shine. It benefits everyone around you and humanity as a whole. If we all practiced this, the world would be a very different place.

While I wrote this book, I remembered days with the Light Beings, even though they occurred a long time ago. I wondered if I could call those same Light Beings in, and to my surprise, when I did, they came. It brought tears to my eyes. It may be something I return to or not, but please, if you find my story enticing, please do a practice where you imagine Light Beings in the room with you. Call them in; let yourself become one of them. Be open to the possibilities, as they can only be good.

Light and love are incredibly healing and empowering ,and that is what this book is about. There are so many things we can do in our everyday lives to live more as light and love. We can even repeat the words "light and love" as we walk, saying a word on each footstep. This brings a walking meditation into our everyday lives. Once you begin to access some of your light, try sending it from your heart and out your eyes to a person, a loved one, or someone you sit with. I invite you to explore your own ways of becoming more of the light and love that you are.

I do have to mention the temporary downside, or not-so-pleasant side, of light and love. We are human beings, and the light will always shine on our darkness. Over the last twenty-five years of meditation, there has been a definite pattern for me, and it slowly changed with probably eighty or ninety percent light and love and ten or twenty percent darkness. I consider the darkness to be when I meditate and am in touch with and healing difficult wounds, feeling all the emotions that were repressed and move through me. Sometimes, the darkness is so difficult that it is all I can say to myself to just take one more breath – just one more breath. It brings tears to my eyes as I remember everything that I healed and how many times it was hard and scary. I often didn't even know what I was healing, but I let the repressed emotions move through me. I remember crying, doing my best to maintain a full breath because it is the full breath that carries the emotions out of us. A full breath processes emotions completely so we never have to do it that way again.

In this way, we can change the past through healing. It would often seem that I would go through periods of slight to intense healing meditations for days or sometimes even weeks, and then I would move into the heights of light and love and even spiritual ecstasy. During those high times, it felt as if those moments would last forever. This was my true self, and it was beyond fantastic. However, then the darkness came again with another more difficult wound to heal, with more repressed emotions to move through me. It often felt like hell, and this is how it goes. We get to the light and it shines on our darkness. If we can endure those times of darkness, we will get to the light again, and over time, our times of light last longer and the times of darkness are shorter. It is always necessary and beneficial to have support when doing this kind of spiritual work. A coach or teacher is ideal, someone who has been through it and became the person you aspire to be like or even be close to. A community is helpful. I would be honored to support you through your time of healing and empowerment.

You deserve to shine in your own and beautiful way. Thank you for taking the time to work with your own light and trust that it is helping your neck issues and your throat chakra. You are worthy of expressing who you truly are and moving forward pain-free. Please feel my support; let it in. Try to receive it into your heart and let my light shine with yours. We are all connected and part of the One Love and Light.

We will now move onto some intensive throat chakra healing. We have done a lot of foundational work to help make the throat chakra healing more effective and to make it more lasting. We want to be able to hold the changes and healing and developing the lower chakras contributes to the change we want to feel in the throat chakra.

Chapter 11:

Intensive Throat Chakra Healing and Development

"Life will give you whatever experience is most helpful for the evolution of your consciousness."
—Eckhart Tolle, *The Power of Now*

Finally, here we are at the chapter you have likely been waiting for. This is where we are going to look at and work intensely with the throat chakra, and we are going to begin by getting a little more intimate with it. Before we do that, however, I encourage you to call in your spiritual support and ask specifically for support and help with healing and developing the throat chakra. Take some time to do this. You may even want to spend time tuning into the heart and throat chakras of the beings who support you, noticing any strengths or characteristics that you are developing or would like to develop in yourself. Remember, everything is already in you. The strengths that you are able to tune into in the beings who support you already exist in you; you just need to uncover them to let these strengths shine.

Preparing for Throat Chakra Healing

Now, before we move into the intense throat chakra, I just want to check in and see how much change you experienced in the first four chakras. These chakras need to be in relatively good shape for the work in the throat to hold well.

Root Chakra

I talked a lot about safety, which is developed in the root chakra. Please continue to do the meditations on bringing light and love into each chakra. You can spend a day or a month on one chakra, but to me, the most fundamental work is creating safety and stability in the first. Go back into the chakra and do your best to heal your inner child before you were five to seven years old. Healing can absolutely be deep and profound, even if you don't have any memories. We all have physical sensations and emotions. This is how the body and heart express the wounds. If it's important that you know what happened, the memory will come. Breathe into physical sensations and emotions, and if the body tenses or wants to move, please allow all of it. Often, the body needs to move, tense, relax, and respond to the work you do in order to release the wounds or trauma that it holds at a cellular level. To take the healing a step further, try to re-parent the little you. Imagine holding the little you and love and cherish that little one in whatever ways that child did not feel loved

133

or cherished. Eventually, even our parents heal when we do this. When I breathe into my root, I now imagine my parents as they are today and how much they love me (even if they don't express it in all the ways I would prefer). As a healed adult, I begin to look beyond the person and feel into my heart.

If you don't feel any love from your parents at this stage of your life, and you have done some healing, it's okay. Sometimes, this love is just so covered over by your parents' wounds and fears that they can't access it at all. Try to imagine it is there, and open your heart to it. After I heal with light and love in the root chakra, I find it useful to imagine my parents as they are today, parenting me back then. I often go back to being an infant and feeling them holding me in their arms, standing close together, looking at me with sparkly eyes, and feeling so much love for me. It may feel like a fantasy, but something transforms within me. I breathe the light and love into all three of us for some time with the intention that not only am I healing the little me but I am also healing my parents. We could all use some healing, so why not include our parents! In the root center, we want to develop a sense of being grounded and of stability and safety, whatever that looks like for us. I love it when clients leave after a healing session with their feet feeling heavier than ever and more grounded than they could have imagined. I wish the same for you!

Sacral and Solar Plexus Chakras

We can move to the sacral and solar plexus chakras in this way, focusing in the sacral on creativity, sexuality, proliferation, and any physical or emotional ailments associated with the sacral. I am not going to provide a list of physical ailments or organs associated with the chakras because I have followed others' advice in the past, and at times, they were wrong. You know your body and your being better than anyone. I encourage you to explore what physical ailment or organ, body part, etc. is associated with which chakra. I mentioned a few qualities of the sacral chakra, and again, please explore your own and heal what you can with love and light. These qualities rise up to the throat chakra where they are expressed or not expressed.

To me, the solar plexus chakra is about truth and power. We find the truth of who we truly are through the solar plexus. In other words, truth is personal power. How can we express who we truly are if we aren't in touch with that or don't even know?

I find so many people with throat chakra issues who have issues with truth and power. You can heal these issues in the solar plexus chakra by breathing in the light and love and again, breathing with the full, rhythmic breath into any and all sensations, emotions, or memories. Try to remember that light and love heals all and that it is your divine right to live in truth and personal power; it is your divine right to express it! You can set the intention that you heal to uncover your personal truth and power. It's all in there and is just waiting to be revealed. Once we discover who we truly are in the solar plexus chakra, we can begin the express it in the throat, which we will learn further on in this chapter.

Heart Chakra

Consider the heart – the ever-so-important chakra and by far the most powerful of all. From Puran Bair, I learned that the pulsed electromagnetic field of the heart is ten times greater than the pulsed electromagnetic field of the brain – what an organ! We can never spend too much time on the heart center, and because you can develop your heart immensely, allowing it to become the light and love that you are while meditating, you can also breathe this energy into any of the chakras, any pain, discomfort, or any illness in your body. You just simply exhale its energy to the location.

Are You Ready?

The more healing meditations you do on the lower centers before moving to the throat, the better. However, please do not expect to completely heal any one or all of the first chakras. I find that healing is ongoing, and we go through different phases. If you moved through at least one or two good healing meditations in each of the first chakras, feel free to move onto the throat. It will likely take more than one practice to have a couple good healing meditations. Be patient with yourself, and don't rush. It is worth spending the time and may take a few tries, maybe even up to a couple weeks. Please take as long as you need to begin by exploring the throat chakra in more detail.

Throat Chakra

What is the color and shape of your throat chakra? What is your throat chakra's temperature? Get intimate with it. Consider the spinning, movement, sensations, and emotions.

136

Don't just necessarily follow me; instead, follow your own guidance. Here is a meditation you may want to try out, even more than once. The intention here is to help you become more familiar with your throat chakra and the entire neck area and what exists for you there personally.

Throat Chakra Meditation

Let's sit nice and straight and lift the head up to the cosmos, feeling the feet firmly on the floor and the seat in the chair. Open the body and heart to the breath by lifting the shoulders way up and stretching them far back, then letting them fall and relax. Feel the shift in the chest and heart center. Take on the full breath and slowly make it rhythmic. Ask or open to your spiritual support. As mentioned before, it is ideal to begin by inhaling love and light from front and back into the heart chakra and exhaling all that love and light into the heart chakra. By working with this chakra first, we feel more energized and uplifted to work with the others. If any difficult physical sensations, emotions, or memories come up for you, stay with them until you have healed them.

Keep doing this, allowing the heart to expand on every exhale. Once you feel your heart is fully expanded, we will move right on to the throat chakra. You will begin the same way, by inhaling love and light from front and back into the throat chakra and exhaling all that love and light into the throat chakra. Placing all your attention into the location of the very center of the throat chakra, breathing into it, ask the throat chakra to show itself, to expose all that is there. You can ask, in your own words, and express your desire a few times, and then just wait, continuing to breathe in the same manner. It can be hard to wait. Whoever says they are fond of waiting?

It can be a bit of a challenge, but we have the breath to focus on while we are waiting, and we can wait with curiosity. You can also ask, 'What would you like to reveal to me?' And wait again. Pay attention to anything that comes, big or small, any colors or shapes, a temperature, a movement of any sort, sensations, emotions, words, dark spots, and just try to stay with it. Make a mental note of what comes, or feel free to stop and write it down, returning to the meditation.

Then we want to enlarge our focus to the greater area of the throat chakra and neck. Include the atlas or spine, the thyroid, the actual throat, etc. See if you can eventually explore the entire neck. Notice what is all there. Ask the neck to reveal anything hidden that would be useful for you to be aware of. Just wait and allow things to come up without ruling out anything. If you think you are making it up, you are not.

Lastly, please expand your focus and breath to include the base of the skull, the ears, jaw, mouth, and chin and down to the shoulders and collarbones.

Continue to breathe light and love into this much larger area, and notice what your body and being reveal to you. At any time, if something comes up that needs to be healed, please seize the opportunity and stay with it, breathing love and light into whatever it is. I encourage you to do this meditation multiple times, or until you feel you have accessed and healed all you can. It is beneficial to repeat this meditation once a month, just to see where it is and if there is anything else that was previously hidden in the subconscious that wants to heal now.

This exploration is valuable in that it gives us much needed information and insight as to our current condition. It can help us understand the wound(s) that are the source of our pain and the source of what holds us back in life. Now, I hope this meditation of exploration helped you to develop a list of areas that need improvement in the throat chakra. I never had such a list and wish I did. I worked on the throat chakra for years and wasn't entirely aware of all that I tried to heal. I had a lot of neck pain, and I wanted that to be gone. I didn't look at a whole lot of other symptoms other than realizing I had trouble expressing myself. When I look back, I see that my list was long. I will just share what I remember now in the hope that it helps you connect more deeply with symptoms that might be true for you. I cannot possibly cover all the wounds held in my throat chakra over the years, let alone all the possible wounds in the throat chakra of everyone reading this book, but here is a list of some:

- Canker sores in childhood and early adulthood
- Sore neck
- Pinched nerve in neck
- Sore shoulders
- Laryngitis through twenties until divorce
- Shy and mousy
- Emotionally disempowered
- Tonsillitis
- Hypothyroid
- Feeling unseen
- Feeling unheard
- Hearing loss
- Grinding teeth from infancy until I started meditating
- Tinnitus
- Feeling disempowered
- Feeling criticized
- Lack of faith
- Difficulty making decisions
- Playing small (big issue)
- Giggled instead of talking as a child; nervous and didn't know what to say
- Couldn't speak up in groups at all
- Neck injuries
- Serious lack of discernment
- Immune system problems
- Fear of expressing my personal truth and power
- Feeling misunderstood
- Depression

When I wrote this list, it was the first time that I'd ever recognized the work I did as I healed almost everything on this list completely, and I know I am well on my way to healing them all completely. I hope you find this encouraging, and I can promise I can help you heal your list much faster than it took me to heal mine.

Please continue to do the first meditation in this chapter, further exploring the throat chakra. Look for any and all energetic wounds that arise from not expressing your truth or your true self. Look for any subconscious memories of dysfunctional ways you expressed yourself over the years and any dysfunctional ways you seek approval and express yourself inappropriately. See if you can see a thread that runs through the patterns. What event is the pattern rooted in? Whatever you uncover, you can heal with love and light on the breath, and then you can create new patterns that serve you so much better. How does your throat chakra want to express what is in your heart now? What are the words your heart and throat chakra would like you to use now that you didn't use before? Create your own personal meditations. You deserve it. Please give yourself the time to heal the wounds that cover your light. Remember to love and nurture the younger you in any way they come up in memories. Give your throat chakra a chance at a new beginning to express authentically.

Express Truth and Power Through Throat Chakra

The expression of your personal truth and power through the throat chakra further is definitely healing, but that true expression also empowers the throat chakra. All the teaching and coaching I do and all my own meditations are based on healing and empowerment. Energetic healing is like cleaning house or weeding a garden, and empowerment is like living in a sparkling clean house or blossoming like a beautiful garden. We want to do as much as possible in the healing phase, and then we move into empowerment, so know that there is light at the end of this tunnel. The following is a practice that can change everything, and we need to first spend the time, as suggested earlier in this chapter, to explore the third chakra and begin to uncover what is true. Once you feel ready for this practice, begin to meditate and set the intention that you are going to bring all that is true in the solar plexus chakra up to the throat chakra and express it. This is so exciting, and it's a moment I've been waiting to enjoy with you.

Truth and Power Meditation

Get into your posture and take on the full, rhythmic breath. Imagine all the spiritual support you have surrounding you, and tune into their specific positive characteristics in their throat chakras. Take a few moments to feel their support and care.

Next, breathe light and love into the heart chakra until it expands. Please take your time, as we never want to rush any of these practices. Once the heart expands with light and love, inhale light and love into the back of the solar plexus to a count of eight (use your melody of "love and light") and hold it there for a count of eight.

Next, exhale the love and light from the solar plexus up to the throat center and forward into the space in front of you (count of eight again). Continue to do this for five to fifty breaths. Then, as you inhale the light and love into the solar plexus, focus on your personal truth and/or personal power in the solar plexus on the hold. If you want to hold longer than the count of eight, hold for sixteen, but remember to hold the breath in the abdomen and not in the chest.

*Then, exhale your personal truth and power up to the throat center and forward, feeling the expression. Continue to do this for five to fifty breaths. Do this as long as feels right. It may feel great at first and then start to get very uncomfortable. It may start feeling awkward, jerky, and difficult, and when you keep doing it, it gets easier. This is a practice that heals and empowers, and only your being knows what you need. Your job is to just keep breathing fully and directing the energy as suggested. You keep counting with the words "love and light" unless you are guided to change them. Maybe you want to breathe "truth and power." Try that or any other words that feel right for you. Make this **your** meditation.*

I discovered I had some wounds of betrayal that were located in the back of the throat chakra. In my twenties, whenever I had an intimate conversation with my ex-husband and told him personal things, he usually used it against me later to belittle or criticize me. Eventually, I stopped sharing with him in these ways, and it made it difficult, if not impossible, for me to share intimately in other relationships until I healed this wound of betrayal.

In the same way, notice anything at the back of your throat chakra, or if you experienced a similar betrayal, look for its location in your throat chakra. Once you locate it and you are meditating, you can inhale the love and light from the back of the center, hold it in the location of the betrayal wound, and then exhale it forward.

Remember when I told you that I had someone on a personal retreat who discovered the whole universe was in her solar plexus? The truth be told, God is in all of our chakras; God is in your throat chakra. I remember when I discovered this. I focused intently in my meditations on the throat, and one day, I saw a small dark spot in the middle of my neck, the front of the actual chakra. I kept breathing love and light into it, and eventually, a spark of light started shining out from inside the dark spot. Continuing with breathing the love and light, eventually the darkness broke up and completely vanished, and I saw, breathed, and felt the light and love of God in my throat chakra. I know this is inside you too; you may not discover it for yourself anytime soon, but I hold the vision that one day you do. In the meantime, I know you can and will heal your throat chakra and feel empowered to express your authentic self in the world the way that is unique in you.

We can certainly ask God for help with this. I'm going to guide you through a meditation in which we let the head drop forward, exposing the back of the neck. Please do not do this practice if it hurts in any way at all. If it begins to feel uncomfortable, just lift the head for a while, still breathing into the throat chakra, and then drop the head again and continue. This practice helps us let God wash our throat chakra. When we feel that all this healing is just too much for us, we can ask for help; we can let God do it for us.

Washing the Throat Chakra Meditation

Sitting in a straight posture with your palms in your lap facing upward to receive, set the intention that you are going to let God (or Source, or the Universe) wash your throat chakra with light and love.

Take on the full, rhythmic breath and breathe light and love into each center three times, starting with the root. When you get to the throat chakra , stay there and continue to breathe light and love. Then, in your own words, ask God for help; make your honest plea. Be specific or general, and trust that your request is perfect for you. Then, in surrender, let your head fall forward, keeping your back straight. Inhale a stream of light and love down from the cosmos into the back of your neck and throat chakra. Exhale this stream into the throat chakra, allowing it to cleanse it. This practice especially helps with wounds of betrayal, but wash whatever is there, any energetic wounds of not expressing your true self and dysfunctional ways we subconsciously seek ap-

proval and any distorted ways we express. If you are aware of what is there, great, and if nothing comes, that is perfect too.

Do this as long as it feels comfortable, then raise the head. Open yourself and your throat chakra to receive, surrendering, allowing all the love and light of the cosmos to wash your throat chakra.

You can continue this surrender with the head up straight by breathing from above into the crown and down into the throat chakra. Continue to exhale into the throat, filling it up. When it feels right, drop your head again and still breathing fully, receive the light and love of God into the throat. Continue with your head down and then up until it feels complete.

Before you stop completely, take some time to ex-hale down through all the chakras to the root for a few breaths and then go further still, exhaling to the center of the earth. The inhale is coming down from the Universe and the exhale goes straight to the center of the earth. This connects us deeply with the earth and the heavenly spheres.

Congratulations on completing the Intensive Throat Chakra Healing. My hope is that you come back here as frequently as you like. You have explored and assessed your throat chakra and what it is there for you personally. Your throat chakra is unique to you just like you are a unique soul in a unique human body. You explored and worked with truth and power and your expression of truth and power and have continued the healing of the throat chakra through washing it with love and light from the cosmos. I hope you are feeling hopeful and renewed.

Chapter 12:

Heart-Centered Shamanism

"Humans are a part of creation and shamanism is our way of connecting with the whole."
—Will Adcock

This chapter is so precious to me, and I hope it touches you in some small or great way. Heart-centered shamanism is something I came up with a number of years ago, as it came to me naturally and unexpectedly. I want to write a book on it one day, so I guess I will start out with a chapter.

I told you my story about how I sacrificed shamanism for Heart Rhythm Meditation. I learned that leaving my body to do spiritual work was not something I wanted to continue to do. I had been doing upward meditation in India and never really liked transcendental meditation because you leave your body. Then, I discovered I could lead a more fulfilling life and experience more happiness with what Puran and Susanna Bair define as downward meditation.

Upward meditation is a spiritual practice designed to draw energy or one's spirit upwards, lifting one's consciousness out of the body. That is where the term out-of-body experience is used. Downward meditation draws energy and one's spirit and consciousness down into the body. I remember meeting a woman who did so much upward meditation that she put rocks in her pockets to try to get herself into her body. To me, downward meditation is most beneficial because your soul or spirit came to earth through this human body to accomplish something. Your soul has always been without a body and will be without a body again. We don't need to do that while we are here. The soul goes on forever. By keeping my consciousness and my soul in my body, I give it more opportunity to fulfill its purpose here on earth.

Over time, even though I practiced downward meditation, my Power Animals would at times come to me, and I would heal and grow in ways I believe I couldn't otherwise. Sometimes, I felt like I was being bad because I was not following the guidelines of Heart Rhythm Meditation, but I always forgave myself, as my Power Animals showed such a keen interest in my very best interest, helping me with goals and parts of myself I wished to improve.

Traditional Shamanism

I learned and studied shamanism through various shamanic teachers and books and even cassette tapes (dating myself here). I also learned how dangerous it can be after I met a couple shamans in Costa Rica who taught me from a distance through the spiritual realms and ended up making me sick because I wouldn't give up my old shamanic ways. I had read about the Bri Bri shamans while in Costa Rica and arranged a guided trip to meet the tribe, see how they lived, and most importantly, meet the shaman. They were brothers. I was able to ask a lot of questions of them, and the translator did a good job of translating their answers. I kind of wanted to stay and learn more from them, but I was part of a small group, and we had to go. When I arrived home from that trip, one of them started to guide me in my meditations through the ethers. Yes, I was in physically in Victoria, Canada, and they were near inland from Puerto Viejo, Costa Rica. These were extremely powerful meditations, and I was sort of awestruck by what was happening until one day, in a shamanic journey, they burned down the old growth cedar tree that I used to journey to the lower world for years. It was so upsetting. I was starting to feel ill and didn't connect the two. As time passed, I became more and more sick, and it was unlike any other time I had been sick. I meditated on it and realized they were making me sick. Thank goodness a fellow shamanic practitioner was able to help me heal and stop them, all in an hour and a half! Maybe this sounds absolutely crazy to you, but I'm sure that, by now, you see I am not your everyday cup of tea. I am here with the sincerest intention to help you heal, grow, progress, and transform with everything that is written in this book. If you are someone who feels a connection with the natural world or with animals specifically, my wish is that you find something to benefit you on your journey.

To me, traditional shamanism is one of the oldest, if not the oldest, spiritual practice in which one enters into altered states through the beat of the drum (sometimes rattle) and leaves the body to journey to three different spiritual dimensions – the lower world, the middle world, and the upper world. The lower world is where one accesses and works with one's Power Animals (also referred to as Spirit Animals or Totem Animals) to assist one's life here on earth. The upper world is the spiritual realm where one works with spiritual teachers and the middle world is the earthly realm as we know it. Of course, there are details I could write another book on, but my hope is this give you a basic understanding of shamanism.

For years when I practiced shamanism, I journeyed through an opening in the ground at the base of an old growth cedar tree, which I visited frequently on my walks. I would go there in my mind's eye. I journeyed to the lower world and did numerous Power Animal retrievals for myself and others. I journeyed there to the beat of my drum, which I made myself. I began the practice with my favorite rattle from Costa Rica. A lot happened in the lower world, and all the work I did there with Power Animals and other beings helped me feel safer in the world, helped me discover more and more about myself, and pointed me in the direction of where I am now.

Journeys to the upper world were where I would receive help and guidance from spiritual teachers. Journeys in the middle world (where we live) helped me let go of the past and welcome the future. I learned to merge with the spirits in nature – spirits of trees, plants, rocks, and mountains, spirits of all living beings, and even got to be pretty good at shape-shifting. Shape-shifting is where we totally become the other, whether human, plant, or anything in nature. We completely lose the sense of self and take on the other so as to think and feel as the other. When one shape-shifts into an animal, other animals in a natural setting, other animals lose their fear of one as a human and come as close as they would normally. Shape-shifting into tree or plant once was a protective measure to keep wild animals or humans from seeing one in the forest. Merging is the practice to master before shape-shifting. Merging is taking on the other while still being conscious of the self. One is the animal or plant or whatever at the same time one is the self. Shape-shifting and Merging are actually practices where one remains in the body and so, to me, can be very valuable to a certain extent. It is ideal to work with a teacher to make sure you are comfortable and safe. We will be working with merging later in this chapter where you will be encouraged to keep practicing so you can move into shape-shifting. If you are working on your own, please only practice with animals, birds, or reptiles to begin with.

Soul retrieval is a shamanic practice that Sandra Ingerman, shaman, teacher and author, became famous for. I believe it was the first book she published. It is titled *Soul Retrieval,* and it was one of her subsequent books *Medicine for the Earth* that I took with me on my five-month backpacking adventure in East Africa. I admire her for her work. I never trained in soul retrieval, but it started happening naturally when I worked with my clients. Soul retrieval is a shamanic practice designed to mend the fragmented soul. The belief is that often when one experiences trauma, part of the soul leaves in order to survive. This loss of part of the soul shows itself in negative behavior, beliefs, etc. Through the practice of soul retrieval, the shaman journeys to the disconnected or lost part of the soul, retrieving it and bringing it back to the person, allowing them to re-integrate it. It is a pretty serious and intense practice, which I have discovered can still be done by oneself through meditation or through the energy healing that I practice.

Ayahuasca is Not for Me

The ever-growing popular use of ayahuasca is not what I consider shamanism. It may be a spiritual means for some people, but years ago, so was LSD and other drugs. Have I tried it? Yes, out of curiosity since I was in Ecuador in the Amazon Jungle where the plant is grown, and there are numerous shamans to do the ceremony with. Will I ever do it again, or do I recommend it? Not a chance for a multitude of reasons. One is that I developed a great capacity to work directly with Spirit when I want and how I want, and I don't have to throw up (side effect of ayahuasca) to get there. I can start and stop any practice at any time. After practicing shamanism for years with a drum or rattle, I swore I would never try Ayahuasca, but I am glad I did so I know what I am not missing!

Ayahuasca is a plant grown primarily in the Amazon Jungle. The shaman gathers the leaves of the plant, combines it with other plants, creating a spiritual brew over a fire. It is not just a matter of physically making it. It is a spiritual ceremony the shaman performs starting with the gathering of the plants. The shaman works with the spirit of the plant, through blessing and ritual, and then gives it to the participants. The ceremony is always performed in the evening and usually lasts through the night. Its intention is to heal one and help one grow and advance in life. The problem with doing these ceremonies in South America is that the shamans do not understand life in the western world, so when working with and treating people from the west, they often make them sicker than they were in the first place.

John Perkins, author of numerous books on Shamanism including his first, *Confessions of an Economic Hitman*, worked with Shamans in South America, and it changed him and his life for the better. He wanted to help others do the same and began organizing tours for people from the west to South America. I heard from another shaman that all seemed to be going well, but he eventually stopped because sometimes the experience went well and sometimes it didn't. North American shamans were having to work on some of the tourists after their return because of damage that was done from participating in ayahuasca ceremonies. I have the utmost respect and admiration for John Perkins and believe his intentions were with the purest heart.

Why Heart-Centered Shamanism

So, why Heart-Centered Shamanism? And what does this have to do with your neck issues or your throat chakra? I believe everything is inside us, and all we have to do is access it. Every experience I had outside of my body I could have inside; we don't have to go anywhere. Whether we feel it or not, we are all one; we are connected to everything and everyone. It goes beyond connection. We are all One. There are practices that I developed that help you connect to and work with other beings, and all of this can be done inside your body. You don't even need a drum. After all, you have a built-in drum – your heart! You can journey to the deepest parts of yourself and access whatever you want to the beat of your heart. When I used to journey outside my body, I used my drum and tried to match the heartbeat of the earth. I am bringing Heart-Centered Shamanism into this book because these practices are designed to help you heal and empower your chakras, most specifically your throat chakra.

I discovered the precise location where we can access our Power Animals and most easily connect to sprits in nature or Spirit in anything. Early on in my journey, I learned that everything has a spirit – every living thing, every inanimate object, every relationship, business, project, organization, club, or religion. Nothing exists without Spirit, and we can work with any spirit that we want to work with.

When I had my interior design business, I sometimes journeyed to a design or renovation project to gain a better understanding of what was best for the client. I had some clients – I'll call them Jane and Tom – who moved from their home in another province. I was hired to renovate and re-decorate their new home in Victoria, Canada. I also did a bit of other spiritual work with Jane. They had put their house in Alberta on the market, and one-and-a-half years later, it still had not sold. Tom asked if me if I could do anything to help it sell since I was a shaman. I always tried to make it clear to people that I didn't call myself a shaman; I was a student of shamanism. Now, I might say shamanic practitioner.

I journeyed to the house and kept seeing a row of trees at the back of the backyard that were going to be cut down, and Jane was extremely upset about it. I knew something had to be done about this situation because it was Jane's attachment to the trees that prevented the house from selling. I looked in the kitchen and was guided to tell them where they could place a talisman to help the house sell. It was on the back of the fridge, which was at the center of the house and therefore in the heart of it.

After my journey, I called my clients, and Tom answered the phone. I asked him if there was a row of trees at the back of the house, and he kept replying no. I told him I saw a row of tall, narrow trees at the back of the house and then asked if there were ever a row of trees at the back. He said yes, and they were on the neighbor's property. A few years prior, the neighbor cut them all down, and Jane was extremely upset; she never got over it. Once I heard that, I worked with Jane to help her get over the loss of the trees, and the house sold in five days to a lovely young family. Today, I discovered how I can do all of that within my body.

So, why do we want to stay in our bodies and not leave the body, and what does all that mean? As I said earlier, I'm not one to give you the science. I believe that we are souls that are born into a human body to have a human experience. Our souls have spent a great deal of time not in human bodies, and once the body dies, the soul will spend a great deal of time not in a human body. Your soul came into your body to have a human experience. It knew what it was getting into, and your body is part of your soul's opportunity to evolve. All of our pains, trials, and tribulations are opportunities for your soul to evolve. Working with Power Animals through Heart-Centered Shamanism has made a huge contribution to the healing and empowerment of me and my clients' throat chakras. I will present some of my favorite practices working with Power Animals and encourage you to work with any Power Animals that come to you or feel appropriate.

So, you may want to know how to get your Power Animal. I am going to save that for another book, or you can work directly with me to do that because accessing your personal Power Animal(s) would be an excellent pursuit once you are finished with the process in this book. In this book, I will teach you how to work with specific Power Animals and other beings to help your throat chakra heal and evolve. Everything we do will be through meditation, and we will remain in the body.

Working with Power Animals

Once, while working on my throat chakra with Heart-Centered Shamanism, an Ostrich came to me for the first time to help me specifically with my throat chakra. I have acquired a number of Power Animals that I have worked with over the years and am always grateful for the existing Power Animals that stay with me and always celebrate the times a new Power Animal comes to work with me. Ostrich for me is very much about bringing the heavens or the cosmos down to earth. I have a canvas print on my wall of Ostrich with its head slightly above a small cloud and its feet strongly planted on the earth. It is a bird that does not fly, which relates to me to the soul in the human body. It also has very powerful legs and feet (root chakra), which is what I needed to strengthen to take my seat in doing my work in the world in a bigger way.

Lately, I have been working with Snake and Cobra to help people transform themselves and transform the throat chakra. I will speak more about Snake and Cobra later in this chapter. We will begin by working with Ostrich. Ostrich has a very long and strong neck; quite the throat chakra, wouldn't you say! By merging with Ostrich, we can heal and empower our throat chakras, removing what is blocking us and empowering us to express more of who we truly are. We will work with the qualities of Ostrich in this meditation.

Heart-Centered Shamanism Meditation: Ostrich

> *Sit in the meditative posture and finding your heart-beat, breathe fully. For this exercise, you can count heartbeats with numbers or the word "love," "light," "love and light," or whatever else helps you maintain a rhythmic breath. Call in your spiritual support and feel their desire to help you and support you fully throughout this meditation.*

> *Breathe into and out of your heart chakra from front and back with love and light until it is expanded. Once it is expanded with love and light, breathe into and out of your solar plexus chakra with love and light. When it feels right, please inhale from the space in front of you, through your heart chakra and into the solar plexus chakra at its exact location on*

the inside of the spine. Exhale into the solar plexus chakra, expanding it more and more on every exhale. Repeat this breath several times, focusing intently on the solar plexus chakra.

Set the intention that you access the Power Animal Ostrich through the back of the solar plexus by using the full breath in this way. This is a time to wait and trust that Ostrich will arrive. Wait at every exhale, and eventually, Ostrich will show up. However Ostrich shows up for you is perfect and may be different than how Ostrich shows up for me. For me, the body of Ostrich shows up in the sacral chakra and root chakra. Ostrich has a large body, and I invite you to feel where and how you experience its large body in your chakras. Ostrich has very strong feet and legs. Notice how you experience Ostrich's feet and legs. Try to focus on the strength and power of the feet and legs coming down from the root chakra. Breathe fully into these areas and explore as long as you need.

Of course, there is the very long neck that runs straight up through the heart center, chakra and throat chakra. Breathe into these two chakras to experience the neck of Ostrich. Whatever comes to you is worth paying attention to. How does breathing into the throat chakra of Ostrich help your own chakra. What is Ostrich trying to help you become aware of?

The head of ostrich is in the third eye center. Breathing deeply and rhythmically, focus on the eyes and *the light that is emitted from them. Inhale from the front and back of the third eye chakra and exhale into the chakra, allowing it to expand as you continue to explore the head and eyes of Ostrich. Where do you most experience its mouth, and what does it symbolize for you? Next, you can breathe all of Ostrich, merging yourself with Ostrich so that you feel more of Ostrich than yourself. This may be a constant experience or vacillating. Once you have a strong experience of Ostrich, you can let go of your focus on the chakras entirely. Feel into yourself as Ostrich, and get in touch with the feet, legs, body, the neck, and the head. Keep breathing fully and pay attention to what draws your awareness. Experiment with Ostrich on the breath. How does Ostrich wish to help you with your neck issues? How can Ostrich help your throat chakra shine?*

To me, Ostrich represents a strong connection between the earth and the spiritual realms or heaven. Ostrich can help you move beyond the earthly limited realities and experience a bigger picture – one where you are not only a human, but a soul that has come from the angelic spheres into your body to complete a purpose. Feel your power as Ostrich and what you are here to do in an abstract or specific way.

Snake Power Animal

We can meditate and become much more in tune with the spiritual potential of the throat chakra. We can get a taste of who and what we are becoming. Our spiritual potential is already in there; we are all that, and we just need to discover it. I remember working with Snake for some time, and Snake to me is all about transformation. While we humans shed our skin without realizing it, snakes make it a fantastic ritual. When you want to shed your skin – your old ways – you can merge with snake energy or even become Snake and move into the molting process. I've noticed that I heat up when I do that; there is a warmth I feel emanating from my snake body that releases the old skin that is ready to be shed. For me, it kind of blisters off. I know snakes can be an unattractive creature to many people, but once you take the risk and become familiar with their energy, you will discover much about yourself, including power.

I used to be terrified of snakes – absolutely terrified. My older brother had a pet snake when we were kids, and one day it got out of its aquarium while we were at school. We came home to find my mother on top of the kitchen table waiting for my brother to get home and get his snake. One day, my daughter visited me in Vancouver where we went to the zoo, which houses many rescued animals. I saw a giant albino Burmese python that we were told weighed about 200 pounds – seriously. It was one big and beautiful snake. Its scales were larger than my fingernails and were so smooth and sleek looking that I just wanted to touch them. I actually wanted to hold this snake as close as possible.

I couldn't believe how I felt, as I only ever knew myself to be afraid of snakes. For years, even when I saw garter snakes, I never wanted to get close, even though I was grateful they appeared for me, taking their symbolism at that time of transformation. This is the number one word to me that describes the spiritual symbolism of snake. If you want "transformation," become Snake. Something must have transformed in me through my meditations and/or developing a connection with snake, as I grew to love them.

While the attendant there at the time couldn't let me hold that snake, he invited me into a small back room and let me hold a smaller snake. Yes, I did ask to hold that snake and tried to be persuasive. My daughter was a little embarrassed of her mother's behavior, but she went along with it, especially since she loved snakes her entire life. She's a real animal lover; her first word was kitty – even before she said mama or dada.

When I began the process of writing this book, I called in Snake to help me discover the author within. I wanted to write a book for years and it was an albino Burmese python that showed up. I discovered much symbolism in this particular snake, which helped me take the steps forward that my heart desired. When you work with any Power Animal, I encourage you to put a picture of it or something that represents it in your meditation space or home. I found a photo of that type of python online and printed it off on photo paper and put it where I would see it often, reminding myself of my intentions and what I went through in my meditations. Sometimes, I work with a Power Animal for a long time and get a canvas print made to hang on my wall. This practice applies not only to Power Animals but also to anything symbolic that comes to us in our meditations. We ultimately are the ones to make the choice as to who or what we work with. We are the masters of our own creations and destiny.

To me, working with Snake is a very effective way to create the change we want. It is about shedding the old and becoming the new. This is what we want to do with our throat chakras, and all our chakras, our entire being – shed the old, which is outworn and manifest the new, truer qualities in ourselves, a sort of a rebirthing or resurrection. Are you ready to shed your skin, transform, and experience a rebirth? Please join me in this meditation.

Heart-Centered Shamanism Meditation: Snake

Sitting comfortably in your meditation chair, adjust your body to sit in the ideal posture for meditation. Take on the full breath, making it rhythmic and breathe in this way until it feels natural. Please take all the time you need to set your intention to shed your skin and open your being to that process, however it manifests for you. Calling in your spiritual support, ask for their specific assistance and support in whatever way you feel you need it.

When you feel clear, breathe love and light into each of your chakras two or three times, inhaling the love and light of the whole universe into the chakra and then exhaling this light into the chakra, filling it up and allowing it to expand.

Everything already exists in us, and the transformation through snake already exists. The very back of the solar plexus is where we access the deepest hidden gems. I invite you to breathe into the very back of the solar plexus, tuning into any symbolism with the intention to access all that you are ready to let go of or to shed. Please wait with each breath, allowing the clues to come to you as opposed to seeking them. Snake is never in a rush to shed its skin. Take all the time you need to get a sense of what all exists, all that no longer serves you and is ready to return to the earth as snake's skin.

Once that feels complete, we will bring the cosmos down to earth through the spine. Inhale love and light from the furthest distance in the cosmos, bringing that energy down through your crown chakra and into the back of the solar plexus where you have discovered all that is ready to be shed. Hold the energy of the breath, after the inhalation, with love and light in the back of the solar plexus in its expanded state, holding all that has come to you. Exhale the love and light down the spine and out the root chakra and deep into the earth. Do this about 5-10 times or until you feel your whole spine lit up and you feel ready to become snake.

To become snake, inhale love and light from the cosmos in the same way into the solar plexus, but now, you do not need to hold the breath. Immediately after the inhale, exhale down through the root and into the earth. While you are breathing in this way, allow snake to emerge from the back of the solar plexus and the energy running through the spine. Power Animals are accessed through the back of the solar plexus, so allow it to emerge from there. Keep breathing in this way, focusing on snake, and as it emerges, notice what color snake takes on for you, what type of scales or you may even recognize what type of snake it is. Every type of snake carries a different meaning. Just trust in the process, and let it emerge. What sensations do you experience? Breathe in all the details of what it feels like to be snake.

Once you feel like you have merged with snake or even shape-shifted into snake, breathe love and light into each chakra again, starting with the root chakra. Notice what comes to you in each chakra with you breathing into whatever it is that you are ready to shed through snake. Notice any physical tension or sensations, and if the body needs to move in any way, just let it. Breathe into each chakra until you feel ready to move onto the next.

Now we move into shedding the skin. Breathing love and light into the solar plexus and staying in touch with the whole spine and snake, feel your skin start to loosen or molt. Notice if your body temperature changes to warm or cool. Feel your eyes as snake glaze over. Surrender to the shedding of the skin with each breath. Surrender to the rebirth of your being. You may want to go back to each chakra individually to make sure you are shedding whatever is ready in each of them. When you get to the throat *chakra, don't be surprised if your neck wants to bend forward or back, if your shoulders rise up, or even if your tongue wants to stick out. Trust that whatever happens is serving you and your evolution.*

When all shedding and change feels complete, take time to breathe as the renewed snake with shiny, new skin. Breathe as the transformed you. Let the love and light flow and radiate however it wants to. Breathe the celebration that comes with new beginnings and transformation.

This is a longer meditation and may take a few tries to really get into it or make the most of it. Make this practice your own and following your own intuition.

If you feel like you are in tune with a particular type of snake, you may want to ask for guidance on the specific qualities of that snake or research online. I have typed in the color of certain snakes that have come to me and then researched the spiritual meaning or qualities. I have always found this most helpful, as the universe is always communicating with us, and this is yet another method.

Cobra

Snake comes and goes in my life, but I would like to share with you a little bit about Cobra and how Cobra can help develop the throat chakra. I only recently worked with Cobra when writing this book to work more intently than ever with the throat chakra. Cobra helps so much with the throat chakra because it holds the energy of transformation and also the energy of a widely expanded throat chakra. Snake is very much about shedding the old and allowing the new, which Cobra represents as well, but Cobra helps us empower our throat chakras, making it easy to speak our truth and live our purpose in beautiful ways. To me, Cobra is also very much about being seen – being seen fully. When Cobra sits up and exposes its hood, you can't miss it. It wants to be seen. Cobra will help you find and heal any hidden wound in the throat chakra that secretly doesn't want you to be seen for the amazing person that you are, may not want you to be seen for what you are on earth to accomplish and be. It was through working with Cobra that I was able to access the last bit of the wound in my throat chakra that didn't quite want me to be seen as the spiritual teacher that I am flattened its neck ribs into a hood from my heart center up to my third eye. It was so powerful. I breathed into this hood and felt the energy of Cobra transforming my throat chakra.

One of the fascinating things is feeling the width of this chakra through Cobra's hood. All the work I did was front to back or encircling the entire chakra, but working in this width opened some doors for me and new awareness of who I am and the work I have to do in this world. Cobra helped me access innate abilities in my chakra that I wasn't aware of, which definitely created a greater sense of confidence to write this book and do the work I feel called to do in a bigger way. I could feel my inner ears so strongly and opened myself to hear what I couldn't hear before. I worked through tension in the jaw to help me open up to say all that is important from my heart. Cobra helps us hear and speak our truth.

Once, when working with Cobra for a number of days, the coolest thing happened – I changed from Cobra to King Tutankhamen! I shape-shifted into the gold and blue mask that he wore in the tomb. I could feel the horizontal stripes to represent Cobra's flattened neck ribs, and more doors opened. I had no idea that Cobra was so revered in Egypt. I looked Cobra up online and learned that it is associated with mysticism in at least India and Egypt. Once I did some research, I remembered reading about it in the distant past but was so excited by the revelations I discovered. Some of the qualities that resonated with me around King Tutankhamen was that his mission was to bring life back into balance for the people, and to create the happiness they longed to experience again. The horizontal lines of Tutankhamen speak to me strongly, and further investigation through meditation revealed more symbolism and understanding that the expression of who I am not only needs to be expressed forward but needs to be expressed wide. My work with this book is to help people find their own internal happiness that is not based on events, people, places, or things but on who they are and what they represent and/or their work in the world – an inner happiness that is not subject to anything outside of them. Thank you, Cobra, and thank you, Tutankhamen!

I encourage you to meditate with Cobra following the snake meditation, but work more intensely with the great hood of Cobra and the throat chakra. Let Cobra guide you in discovering qualities in you that want to be healed and/or developed. I encourage you to even meditate as King Tutankhamen if that feels right, and all the characteristics you have in common with him. May you open to Cobra and all the support it can offer in letting your throat chakra shine.

Other Power Animals

I invite you to work with Ostrich, Snake, and especially Cobra and let yourself be healed and empowered through them.

Please don't necessarily stop here. How many living creatures are there in the world and which ones are most beneficial for you to connect with? We have barely touched into working with Power Animals through Heart-Centered Shamanism. I have focused here on the throat chakra, but you may gain a great deal by working with a different Power Animal in another chakra. Often, a lower chakra can really become a catalyst for change for the throat chakra. Work wherever you feel energy is stuck. You can go back to the earlier meditations in this book to assess which chakra is ready for some deep attention and transformation. Please pursue any other creatures you are inspired to practice with using the basics of Heart-Centered Shamanism.

My hope is that you have allowed yourself to be stretched in ways you have never been stretched before, that you have surrendered to accessing qualities in yourself just waiting to be acknowledged and expressed. And really, my hope is that your neck issues have improved and your throat chakra altered in the most positive ways.

Now is the time to move into empowerment. Regardless of where you are at on your journey, you can take this next step into empowerment. We do not have to be completely healed to move into empowerment. I have never really stopped healing, but my healing meditations have become so much less in recent years and the focus has been on being of service through my purpose. You can and hopefully will go back to any of the meditations and even create some of your own. I find it beneficial to stay with one meditation for long periods of time, many days, weeks or even months. Through this approach, we create deeper change and transformation. Some of the practices are meant to be short term and some long term depending on you the individual, where you are at and what you need most. We have been holding the intention of healing our neck issues, and now it is definitely time to let your throat chakra shine in the most beautiful and unique ways.

Let's move into empowerment!

Chapter 13:

Empowerment

*"Who would attempt to fly with the tiny wings of
a sparrow when the mighty power of an eagle
has been given him(her)"*
—Kenneth Wapnick

According to the Oxford Dictionary, "empowerment" is defined as "the process of becoming stronger and more confident, especially in controlling one's life and claiming one's rights." I would like to modify this meaning of the word "empowerment" for use in this book to "the process of becoming stronger and more confident, especially in taking steps toward fulfilling one's life or soul's purpose." That's the kind of empowerment I would like to speak about. You have done a great deal of healing around your neck issues through a variety of powerful practices. You have healed and integrated parts of yourself in surprising and expected ways. This is a pivotal point in this process where we move from healing to empowerment. This is where we move from healing your neck issues to letting your throat chakra shine!

What does empowerment mean to you? What does power mean to you, and how do you apply power and empowerment to your current life? Have you ever been in touch with your greatness? I struggled with stepping into my greatness for way too long, and even though in my mind, I understood it was God's greatness moving through me, when I tried to take steps toward this, I would have a meltdown. I hadn't yet healed all that was getting in my way. I look back now and see that I was in touch with the need in others but wasn't aware of it. The need of others for our service pulls us forward.

Somehow, the universe believed more in me than I could believe in myself at that time. There wasn't anyone around who could help me surrender to this – nobody to hold me in my fear. I felt alone. It was such a difficult time that it made me physically ill, and I became too ill to work. I have been through a few incredibly difficult times in my life, and that was one of them. I came pretty close to dying, and western medicine couldn't help me. It took some time to get myself well again, and I see now how I can help others surrender to their greatness.

What does surrendering to greatness mean? Doing so means letting go of the small self and opening to the true self – the higher self. We cannot do it with the mind, knowledge, or prowess. Instead, we have to get out of the way and let it emerge. To me, it is a passive surrendering. It exists within your being, and this is what I was terrified of. This was the one time I couldn't hold my own fear – the one and only time. I was afraid of what it meant and who I might become, and once I got through it, I realized it was a great fear of being recognized and seen for who I was.

This may not make sense to the logical mind. Of course, we are meant to be recognized for who we are, but in my heart, my wounds of the past prevented this, and it took me some time to move through them. If any of this resonates with you, maybe it's time for you to open your heart and be vulnerable enough to let someone hold you in your fear – hold you in the knowing of who you truly are or what that feels like. Let someone hold you as you move toward that, not knowing how the unfolding will occur. I hope to do my best in this chapter to help you move from being stuck with neck pain and into empowerment.

We worked with light and love in meditation and even Heart-Centered Shamanism to heal what causes neck pain and makes us feel stuck or keeps us stuck. Now we will move toward responding to the need of others for our service. Let's work on surrendering to all that we truly are and more. It cannot be forced with the mind, and this kind of surrender is so powerful that it empowers us. We can surrender to letting God/the Universe in to empower us to be all that we truly are.

Surrender

Have you ever sat and listened to one particular song over and over and cried or felt emotionally moved? I have done this for years and years. One of the songs that I turned to and often listened to in meditation before writing a new chapter in this book was "You Raise Me Up" by Secret Garden. I feel so supported by God when I sing or breathe this song in meditation. The range of tears I shed depends on what I am going through that day or in that particular phase or what is moving through me in life. I breathe into the God in my heart – the God in my heart who raises me up. I think I watched and listened to every single rendition by other artists on YouTube and the version of the song that moves me the most is the original version just like Leonard Cohen's "Halleluiah."

I, as a mortal, cannot stand on mountains, walk on stormy seas, or be more than I can be the way I can with the support of the God within my heart, and it is through surrendering to the love, light, and support of God that I am able to move forward in my life and fulfill my life's purpose. This song gets me in touch with that every single time. It helps me surrender to my humanness and my imperfection, striving for the perfection only within God and allowing that in. I allow it into the most tender and sacred place in my heart and let it fill me up. I listen to this song occasionally for no real reason or when I want that kind of spiritual support, when things are feeling hard and other times when I am feeling on top of the world. Sometimes I meditate, and sometimes I don't. If you don't have a song that moves you, I encourage you to find one.

When I was in the early stages of working on this book, it seemed that everything inside me keeping me from writing this book sooner came up. We all have self-doubt; it's how we move through it that matters. I don't even remember exactly what the struggle was anymore, but I remember the tears I shed through meditation and singing this song over and over. I meditated that morning for over two hours, facing everything that kept me from writing a book, and then I longed to sing this song. I sat at my desk for over two hours and sang this song over and over and breathed it into my heart, wondering if and when the tears would ever dry up.

At that time, I was guiding a very close, long-time friend on a one-week, personal retreat. She had planned to stay in my retreat space in my home, but plans changed, and we ended up doing the retreat online. We would meet on Zoom for one and half hours before sunrise and after sunset for an hour every day to discuss how things were going, and I would give her practices for the following twelve hours. We met that morning, and after breakfast, I meditated. My calendar was clear because I wanted to devote my time to this book. She was doing a retreat on the purpose of her life, and what got in her way started to come up for her. We are all so connected, and I wonder if this helped me get in touch with what was getting in my way of writing this book and becoming more of who I truly am.

Together, we had almost four and a half hours of tears; it felt like it would never end. The tears were far from all sad; I think the last two-plus hours of tears were of the joy from breaking through that which I couldn't break through before. I played this song over and over and felt so beautifully raised up – fully knowing that it was not just me. I was completely and indefinitely supported by God. The tears of joy and gratitude flowed and flowed. The tears moved from fear and trepidation to tears of ecstasy knowing I was going to write a book to make a difference in the world in my own unique way. I didn't know exactly what it was going to all say, but

I was in touch with my purpose, the book, and incredible support I had to let God move through me in divine expression to somehow help others.

When we got on our video meeting later that day, we meditated together briefly, and she asked me what I had done to her. She had maybe half a dozen healing sessions from me in the past, and she told me she felt like I was doing a healing on her for almost four and a half hours and was actually convinced that I sat there all morning doing one long healing session on her. Her schedule was to stop meditating around noon and have lunch, and she couldn't stop. Instead, she meditated until just before one p.m., which was when the tears stopped for me. I remember looking at the time, and it was 12:52 p.m. It was an experience unlike anything else she experienced. She thought it was all me, and I have to wonder who was doing what. This is such a compelling example of how when we heal and grow, others heal and grow. There is some great law in the universe that exists – a law that allows others to heal when we heal, whether it is our intention or whether we know it or not. We really are all one, and when we help ourselves, we help others, and when we help others, we help ourselves. What we experience as separation is an illusion, so the closest people to us benefit from the personal work we do and so do our clients.

So, you can see, this song does a lot for me, and it may or may not do the same for you. I encourage you to meditate and breathe through each word, into and out of your heart and your entire being. If it doesn't evoke that response in you, try to find a song that does and listen to it, breathe it into your heart – your entire being – in meditation and surrender to the sounds, the words, and the energy behind it from which it was created.

Living from Your Deathbed

Another practice that came to me some time ago that I find empowering is "living from my deathbed." I learned to make big decisions by imagining how I would feel about my choices in life from the view of being on my deathbed. This began when I was traveling in Uganda and went to see the mountain gorillas in Bwindi National Park. It was one of the highlights of my life! We were a small group with our guides, hiking in the jungle for a few hours, and the guides cut the way with machetes. We sat with and observed the mountain gorillas for about an hour and trekked out; it was magnificent!

I went up with a few people in a RAV4, and soon after that extremely magical event, we headed down the mountain on a steep, single-lane dirt road with no guardrail, and the brakes failed. The driver pulled the emergency break, and that failed as well. We picked up a lot of speed, and I knew if we didn't slow down, we would go over the edge to a drop over a thousand feet. The driver decided to hit the wall of the side of the mountain to make us stop, and after we clammed head-on into it, the vehicle flew up in the air and landed upside down, rolling four times in total. I thought that was it. I kept imaging the cliff that was so close and how inevitable it was that we would go over it.

After rolling four times, the vehicle landed upside down and slid down the dirt road, caving in on itself. None of us wore seatbelts, and I was upside down with my chin rammed into my chest, the back of my neck taking a tremendous beating. I started to surrender to my impending death and suddenly started to plead and pray, "No God, please save me."

I waited for what seemed an eternity. The vehicle stopped about two feet from the edge of the cliff. People from the vehicles behind us came and pulled us out. After that event, I knew I had lived because I had something in the world to do. It was a deep knowing, and it never left me. I wasn't sure what it was, but I knew beyond a doubt that it was something and it was important for me to discover and live it. This was another great blow to my throat chakra, but sometimes that's what it takes to get our attention.

When I returned to Canada after those five months in Africa, I looked at the personal journal I had not taken to Africa with me. I completely forgot that the last thing I did before I left on that five-month trip was a shamanic journey to the lower world, and it was my Power Animal Gorilla who met me there. I recorded this shamanic journey in the journal and left on my trip that day. I asked for the most important message for me before I flew to Africa. In the journey, I was with Gorilla high up on a mountain, which was a first. I always worked with gorilla in a forest but never on a mountain. At the time, I couldn't believe what happened in that journey with Gorilla, who helped me so much for years. Gorilla repeatedly tried throwing me off the mountain! I was there on the side of the mountain with him, and he would throw me as hard as possible horizontally out into the air, and somehow, I kept pulling myself back to the mountain. I could not make any sense whatsoever of this spiritual experience or get the accurate message in it.

At that time, I hadn't even considered going to see the mountain gorillas in Bwindi, let alone plan that adventure. Was it a warning? Was it a divine plan? This experience reminds me that the universe is always communicating with us, and the more we open to it, the better. Somehow, even though I felt somewhat lost in my life when I returned to Canada, I also felt the beginnings of empowerment developing within me. From that experience, I knew I had something to accomplish – a purpose unique to me, some kind of important work to do.

Brushing up that closely with death immediately gave me a new perspective to live by. Whenever I had a big decision to make, I imagined how I would feel about any of the possibilities from the perspective of being on my deathbed. One of my favorite Rumi quotes is, "Die before you die."

Carl Jung wrote on this subject and a couple of his quotes that resonate with me are, "Shrinking away from death is something unhealthy and abnormal which robs the second half of life of its purpose" and "Your vision will become clear only when you can look into your own heart. Who looks outside, dreams, who looks inside, awakes."

If you can meditate on being on your deathbed and look into your heart at that time, imagining it fully, you will make the best choices for yourself, even if they seem strange to others. You can use this with big decisions and the smallest as well. If you practice this often enough, it becomes a way of living. It can empower you to make the best decisions.

The first spiritual book I ever read was Elisabeth Kübler-Ross's *On Death and Dying*. She worked with the dying in a way that had never been done before, and one of the things she discovered was all the regrets people had about their lives. Regrets are not only felt in the heart but the regrets of not expressing what we are here to express is felt in the throat chakra. Many wished they wore more red or purple clothes, and I wonder if this inspired the Red Hat Society. I am so proud of my mother, who is the Red Hat Queen of the Flamin' Floozies Red Hat Society. These women want to live fully and not have regrets of not doing so. I think this shows possibilities, but what is there more for you? Wearing a red hat may feel great, but what else would you like to do or be so that your throat chakra shines through this life and when you are on your death bed you feel ever so satisfied that your life was so worth living? What is it that you want to be on your death bed feeling happy about? What is it that you will be grateful you accomplished, taught others, or any other expression of your reason for being here? What are your regrets right now that you still have time to become, do, live or be? Of course, meditating on your heart chakra and your throat chakra to discover more of what is waiting to be uncovered is something you can do again and again.

This Meditation involves Pranayama Breathing which I encourage you to practice first so that it flows easily in the meditation.

Basic Pranayama Breathing

Pranayama means expansion or control of the life force. Prana means "life force" or "vital energy," and ayama varies in meaning from control to expansion. It is a practice of controlling the breath to raise one's energy. Pranayama breathing techniques were developed roughly 6,000 years ago by ancient sages of India. I have focused on and practices the various techniques I have learned while in India and in North America and find them especially helpful in certain meditations. Remember, it is the power of the breath that can be most transformative.

We need to block one nostril when practicing pranayama, and there are a few different ways to do this. I prefer the traditional style I learned in India. You can do this by looking at the palm of your dominant hand. Keeping all fingers relaxed and fairly straight, bend the pointer finger, and middle finger forward. Keeping the ring finger and pinkie finger together, let the thumb and two remaining fingers become like pinchers or crab claws. You can now practice blocking one nostril by raising your hand up to your nose and try blocking one nostril and then the other. Your arm won't get too tired if you keep it tucked against your body. You can do this practice on its own, and it does a great job of creating balance within oneself. It is ideal to start with a shorter period of time and make it longer as feels appropriate. In this practice, we hold the breath, but in the next meditation, we will not hold the breath. If practicing this as a meditating on its own, start with seven repetitions and increase by one repetition every two or three days. Please note that in this meditation we start with blocking the right nostril, and in the next meditation, we begin with blocking the left because it serves a different purpose – going back in time.

Basic Pranayama Breathing Meditation

- ◆ Sit on a chair in the Pharaoh posture
- ◆ Block your right nostril, and inhale slowly through the left nostril for six or eight counts (seconds or heartbeats)
- ◆ Block both nostrils and hold your breath in the belly, not the chest, for twelve or sixteen counts
- ◆ Block the left nostril and exhale slowly through the right nostril for six or eight counts
- ◆ Repeat left to right breath above seven times
- ◆ Block your left nostril, and inhale slowly through the right for six or eight counts
- ◆ Block both nostrils and hold your breath in the lower abdomen for twelve or sixteen counts
- ◆ exhale through the left for six or eight counts
- ◆ Block the right nostril and exhale slowly through the right nostril for six or eight counts
- ◆ Repeat right to left breath above seven times
- ◆ Place your hand down and inhale through both nostrils for six or eight counts
- ◆ Hold the breath in the lower abdomen for twelve or sixteen counts
- ◆ Exhale through both nostrils for six or eight counts
- ◆ Repeat both nostril breathing above seven times

Deathbed Meditation

Please take your seat in your chair and just notice where your normal breath is, what emotions, thoughts, or physical sensations you notice, if any. Just sit for a few minutes and be with yourself exactly as you are in this moment.

When it feels right, make the breath full and then rhythmic. For this meditation, you can use the words "love and light" to maintain your rhythm with the breath, or you can just stay with the melody or use numbers to count heartbeats or seconds. This is a fairly intense meditation, so do whatever works best for you.

Please call in your spiritual support.

Begin with pranayama breathing, which is described above.

For this practice, we will not hold the breath at all.

Your intention here is to make discoveries about your life, in the past, present and future, which can contribute to the further healing of our neck issues and empowering the throat chakra to make it shine. View your life from our deathbed so that you can make the best decisions for yourself today.

Please put your hands in the position described earlier and block the left nostril, inhaling for a count of six or eight from the furthest distance you can imagine on the right, and then block the right nostril and exhale out the left nostril to the furthest distance on the left.

Continue to do this breathing from right to left with the intention of going back in time. Keep inhaling from the right and as you exhale left, go back until you are ten years younger than you are now. Allow any memories, emotions, or awarenesses of what has significantly contributed to your neck issues or throat chakra health. Go there on every exhale to the left until you have some sort of information.

Continue in this fashion the same way until you are twenty years younger than you are now. Again, allow whatever wants to come up to come up. Continue exhaling to the left until you go back to your time of birth. How has your birth contributed to who you are today? Wait for any emotions or memories to surface and breathe into whatever presents itself. Continue on only when this feels complete.

When it feels right, please reverse the breath by blocking the right nostril and inhale in through the left nostril and then exhale out the right while blocking the left. Continue to breathe in fashion until you come back in time to the present. Take as many breaths as you need, as there is no rush.

Once you have returned to the present, we will continue breathing from left to right until we are ten years in the future. This usually takes longer than going back in time, so keep breathing until it feels like you are ten years older. Allow the future events, situations, or awarenesses to come to you based on the changes you are experiencing in your neck and throat chakra. Stay there, allowing and breathing in all that comes to you. Continue to go forward in time, inhaling from left to right until you are twenty years older than you are now. Again, allow all that wants to be presented to you to come. Stay there until you have the information you need, and take the time to breathe into it, to integrate it into who you are now. Continue in this way until you are at your time of death.

Imagine you are on your death bed.

Let yourself look back on your life and notice what you are most grateful for. How has this work on the throat chakra changed your life path in positive ways? Is there anything you could change now that would contribute to a deeper sense of gratitude and completion on your death bed? What would that be? What kinds of emotions do you want to feel on your deathbed? Give yourself all the time you need. Breathe deeply into whatever comes. You can create any changes you want in your life now, from this perspective.

Once this feels complete, change the breath to inhaling from the right and exhaling to the left until you are back in present time, in this exact moment.

*Breathe into your root chakra and ground yourself
well into the earth.*

I encourage you to write in your journal all that came to
you. Based on what came to you in your meditation, how do
you want to live your life differently? What changes do you
wish to make and when? It is important to pay close attention
and follow the guidance you received in this meditation. It is
ideal to take at least one action step as soon as possible after
this meditation. Let this meditation and what you gain from
it empower you to make the changes you desire in yourself
and in your life. And if you received specific guidance around
the empowerment of your throat chakra, follow that as soon
as possible! When we take an action step, it gets the energies
of change flowing in the right direction. The more action
steps we can keep taking, the better. You may have fear or
resistance come up, but you can meditate on it or just take
Susan Jeffers's advice and "feel the fear and do it anyway!"
So, please make sure you write down everything that came
to you and create a list of action steps and follow them as
soon as you are able.

Because of the intensity of this meditation, most people
can only practice it once in a while and not every day. Don't
feel you need to do it every day like the earlier practices
unless you love doing it.

The practice you can do every day based on this meditation is to make the daily decisions in your life based on how
you want to feel on your deathbed. Whatever decisions you
need or want to make, ask yourself, how will I feel on my
deathbed if I choose the first option, and how will I feel on my

deathbed if I choose the second option? And, when related to your throat chakra, you can even ask, will my throat chakra be shining brightly at my deathbed if I choose this or that?

In shamanism, I did a number of dismemberment journeys when I was guided to. They were always incredibly intense, yet powerfully transformational. I journeyed to the lower world with the intention of dying to be born again. The experience was difficult to stay with as one becomes dismembered by an animal, or like in one dismemberment journey, I was burned at the stake and was then reborn with the elements of earth, fire, water, and air from the ashes in an unexplainable way.

I could lead you on a meditation for this purpose in this book, but I believe this is something best done in person or at the very least on a video or audio recording. It is certainly something you can reflect on and work with yourself. Spend some time in meditation imagining yourself on your deathbed and who in your life now means a lot to you and how you would feel about the relationship and your behavior when you die. I find that this practice helps me forgive others more quickly and easily because it helps me quickly get in touch with love and teaches me the importance of the love and remaining in love as much as possible. I want to be on my deathbed having written this book. It gives me the courage and helps empower me to follow the knowing that this book was something worth completing, regardless of how difficult it was.

I would like to lead you in one of many empowerment meditations. Please continue to do this regularly and alter it to better suit you and your purpose, whether you are aware of what that is or not. I invite you to first reflect on a few questions and make notes in your journal:

- How have you expressed well in your life to date?
- What is calling to be expressed through you in your unique way?
- What is the need in the world that waits for you to fulfill it?
- What is the great need in certain individuals that is just waiting to hear your message, receive your service(s), or work with you in some way?
- What is pulling your heart forward?
- Who needs what you have to offer?
- What does Source, God, the Universe want to express itself through you? How do you, or can you, create the space for that?
- What is the biggest message your heart would give you today if it could?

Thank you for doing your best to answer these questions. Now through meditation, let'ssee what further truths you can access in your chakras, the truths that are waiting to be expressed in your throat chakra.

Purpose Meditation

Let's get into the meditative posture. Move into the full, rhythmic breath; Take a moment to call in your spiritual support. Remember all the work you have done so far, all the meditations you have done with the chakras, Power Animals, and energy.

Let's begin by breathing into the heart center and expanding it with light and love. Breathe into all that is there, the desire and purpose in your heart. Keep exhaling into your heart, expanding the energetic pericardium until it is beyond your physical form and you are sitting inside your heart chakra. When this experience is constant, starting with the root chakra, breathe light and love into all the chakras, spending more time in the solar plexus, the deep heart. This is where you access your purpose.

As you breathe light and love there, exhale into that chakra and imagine there is a membrane around this chakra as well. Expand that membrane to make the solar plexus much larger, allowing you to access a sense of your purpose even if your mind isn't yet aware of what that is. Fill it with all the love and light of the entire universe. Do the same thing when you get up to the throat chakra, expanding it to be much larger, allowing for a great expression of what is in your solar plexus and heart chakras.

Next, we will go back to the root, and we will imagine our soul coming into being at the back of the root. I invite you to inhale your soul that made the choice to be born into your human form. Inhale that into the tip of the coccyx – this soul that has a great intention. You need a strong root to hold this practice, and you have been working on that. Know your root chakra can accept and hold all that your soul came here for. After the inhale, exhale up to the back of the solar plexus and fill the solar plexus on the exhale. Do that for five to ten breaths. Next, still inhaling from behind the root and into the root, get in touch with the deepest part of yourself – your soul that chose to be born into this world – and exhale that energy up to the heart center and fill the heart center. Do this for five to ten breaths. Next, inhaling into the root again, send this energy up to the throat center, filling it up and letting it expand further. Once you have done this for at least five breaths, let the energy flow out of the throat chakra in all directions, like a fountain, and then after five to ten breaths of that, exhale the energy forward. You are exhaling the expression of your soul's purpose.

When you repeat this practice, try to surrender to the need of others, feeling their need like a magnet pulling from you your soul's purpose. Surrender to this pull and allow God to move through you. This kind of surrender can be very empowering. All the visible and invisible support around you to help and support you in your unfolding. Surrender to your greatness and your unique and specific calling.

I mentioned at the beginning of this chapter my definition of empowerment – "the process of becoming stronger and more confident, especially in taking steps toward fulfilling one's life purpose." And this is a further step in healing your neck issues and a series of steps to letting your throat chakra shine. Thank you for taking the steps and working with the practices in this chapter toward you calling, your purpose. You still do not need to know exactly what that is 100 percent, but my hope is you have some clues, some ideas, and that you have had some aha moments that give you the courage to keep moving forward. The practices are here to continue to use, and know that every time you do them, you are getting closer. Sometimes the practice results in an opening and other times a great epiphany. It is the sitting and doing that practices that will continue to empower you and let your throat chakra shine.

We have taken many steps toward healing, discovery of purpose, followed by steps to empowerment, and now I look forward to taking giant steps toward purpose with you. I have mentioned purpose many times and believe we are all on a path toward purpose without even knowing what it is. The knowledge of our specific purpose often comes after we have been living it without necessarily knowing it.

Chapter 14:

Giant Steps toward Purpose

"Faith is taking the first step even when you don't
see the whole staircase."
—Martin Luther King, Jr.

I could have named this chapter "Steps toward Purpose,"
but I have been one of these people who has the attitude of,
"Go all the way or go home!" Let's go all the way together. You
began with this book in small steps, and those steps steadily
increased in degree. Now, let's take some giant steps. You
became used to facing and feeling your fears and took steps
to move beyond them. Now is the time to put the pedal to
the metal if you so wish.

Where is your neck pain? Is it lingering or completely
gone? Is it old pain, new pain, or has the pain moved elsewhere? Please take time to assess this and continue to practice the meditations provided in this book.

In this chapter on giant steps toward purpose, you want
to be in touch with all bodily sensations not only in the neck

but also in the entire body. You also want to be aware of your emotional state as well. When you begin to take steps forward toward your purpose, whatever was holding you back in the past will begin to come up. Yes, you have likely healed a lot of that, and that is why you are at this point, and that is why you are willing to keep going.

Personally, taking steps forward sometimes feels like an emotional roller coaster. I begin to take steps that my heart longs for, and it feels amazing; I feel like I'm on top of the world and trust everything will be fine – until it isn't. Have you ever experienced anything like this?

Stepping forward involves *risk*. It is never comfortable. If it were comfortable, it wouldn't be risk. Our human conditioning is that of survival, and doing something new and different does not ensure survival. Fear of some sort is going to come up, occasionally or frequently. Please remember Susan Jeffers and feel the fear and do it anyway. I wish it was always that simple.

To me, there is another step to this to ensure that exact same fear doesn't come up again, and that is through meditation. For years now, when I feel the fear, I move into meditation and allow myself to feel that fear fully; the fear leaves me, and I can proceed, but other times, it keeps coming up, or I don't quite get through it. This is where you need to do more work. You need to heal your past, and meditation can help you get there. My experience is that even when I think I completely healed a childhood wound and it hasn't come up for many years, it may reappear at a deeper level right when I am in the midst of taking a giant step forward. For example, this happened to me once when I wrote this book. I had to heal wounds I already healed, but the wounds wanted to be healed at a deeper level. I couldn't have faced this before because I never tried to write a book before. As I mentioned earlier, it took two hours of meditation, and then I celebrated with a song for two hours, but I got through it. That morning, writing this book went from extremely difficult to a most enjoyable flow, and it never went back to being difficult again. Any process that changes us and helps us access and bring out who we truly are in the world is usually going to be challenging, and this is one of those processes. Please keep doing the meditations and trust that everything is perfect, exactly as it is, even when stuff comes up.

Purpose

What is your purpose? This is, in my opinion, one of the most difficult questions to answer in one's life. I remember talking to a young British fellow about purpose when I traveled in South America. At that point in my life, I was searching. That is why I travelled for twenty months, and all I came up with was that my purpose was something. I could sort of feel it in a concrete way, yet it was obscure. I didn't know exactly what it was, but I somehow knew I was meant to help others. The British fellow had given up; he believed that it was a question everyone eventually asks but that the majority of people will never know, so it is best to stop asking and forget about it. We had quite the discussion and agreed to disagree.

Where do you currently stand on this subject? Do you feel a desire to help others? I believe this is one indicator that you are getting closer to your purpose. I invite you to feel into that knowing when you meditate on your chakras. Call in your spiritual support, and attune to this as much as you can. Breathe in the light and love and then breathe that knowing of helping others into each chakra. You can even change the words from "love and light" to "helping others," using the words "helping others" to count your heartbeats as you inhale, hold the breath, and exhale. Be open to what your being wants to tell you. Accept whatever happens in any particular chakra as a message.

Is there still something holding you back, and is it presenting itself by physical tension or pain, or does the chakra light up or feel energized? What kinds of emotions surface? Do any memories suddenly come up? Whatever it is, breathe through it. Maybe you are closer to your purpose than that; maybe you know you are a healer of sorts, but you are not exactly sure what that specifically looks like. On the other hand, maybe you are a healer of sorts, and you know that your purpose is to develop that to another level so you can help others more than you already are. Wherever you are and whatever your heart's desire is, bring that into your meditations and into each of the chakras, one at a time. At this point, if you discover anything new in any of the chakras that needs to be healed, I invite you to spend as much time there as required until you return to the feelings of light and love. Let the light and love fill every chakra and your entire being. Breathe it in like a sponge – receive, receive, receive. If anything came up from early childhood, take that little you, and love that little you like they have never been loved before. Nurture and love with words, gestures, or holding in the ways they deserve to be loved.

Maybe you know exactly what your purpose is. Perhaps your purpose is as clear as day and you hope that one day you can fulfill it, but now is not the time. I discovered that it actually hurts us to refrain from fulfilling our purpose once we know it. I discovered my purpose and became ill when I resisted it and did not take steps toward fulfilling it. This is not to instill fear in you and certainly is not a threat, but please pay attention. If you know what your purpose is and you are not taking steps to fulfill it, what else is happening in your life? Often illness, accidents, and mishaps are ways the Universe tells us that we are off track; these are often wakeup calls. In my experience, I could see how the Universe said to me, "What's it gonna take for you to accept the fact that you are a spiritual teacher and start living it?" I wish I knew then what I know now.

Automatic Writing Through Meditation

Next, we want to open to guidance through our heart and our throat chakra. Remember that everything is inside us; we just need to access it. What are your next steps? What are your giant steps toward purpose? Please take some time to reflect on this. See what comes up for you at the level of the mind. Whatever comes to mind immediately, write it down; don't edit or second guess yourself. For work like this, I like to use automatic writing, which I first learned years ago when I was doing the artist's way. *The Artist's Way* is a workbook on creativity, published by Julia Cameron roughly twenty-five years ago. One learns to do automatic writing under the heading of "Morning Pages," which Julia describes as "three pages of longhand, stream of consciousness writing done first thing in the morning." I never did finish that book, but the automatic writing helped me quite a bit for the brief time I did it. I return to that skill when I want access to my inner knowing, and then I meditate on whatever comes to get clarification.

To write, you can use your journal or your computer. I like to sit at my computer, ask the question, and breathe into my heart chakra and then later into my throat chakra. I actually close my eyes and keep breathing into my heart. You can take on the full, rhythmic breath or not – whatever feels right for you. I encourage you to find your own method. Mine is to sit, meditate for ten minutes or longer on the question I ask myself, and then start typing. Please keep your eyes closed as much as possible and let the words flow from the heart or throat chakra and keep your focus on that one chakra throughout this practice. Just type whatever comes, even if it doesn't make any sense, and keep typing until you know you are finished. Don't stop typing if you're not getting anything, just type, "nothing is coming" or whatever feels right until the next piece comes. You will often be surprised by at least one or two things that you write. I suggest to first do this practice focusing on the heart chakra with the intention to discover how you can best follow your heart. Later, try focusing on the throat chakra with the intention on how you can better speak your truth, express yourself, or specifically how your throat chakra wants to shine.

Another method is to ask God through automatic writing. I used to do this method when I used to experience God as outside of me, but now I can find God inside my heart, so that is why I like to focus on my heart chakra. If you do not experience God in your heart yet – just imagine or trust that God is in your heart always as the perfect exercise for you. Write from your heart to God asking for guidance. Write about your feelings, where you are in your journey, and what you specifically want God to answer. You can even pray; do whatever feels right. This is especially useful if you are not sure what your exact question is. A great question to ask God is how amazing, wonderful, and loveable you are! The next step is to write from God's perspective. Imagine you are God or that God is writing through you. First off, God is thrilled that you are asking, and know that God wants to answer your question(s). Close your eyes, breathe into your heart, and start writing as God. Whatever you do, don't stop until it is finished, and your question in answered. It is such a shift in experience to do this, and I would love to hear what this is like for you.

Please use this method of automatic writing through meditation to discover what your actions steps are here. It's great to get guidance in meditation, in healing sessions, or have a knowing of what we need to do, but it is so important to get the energy flowing well, and we do this by taking action steps. After private sessions or a healing, I love to give homework exercises because it furthers the healing and growth. Once you know what your action steps are, schedule them in. If an action step is something that you don't know how to do, create an action step where you do the research to find out how to do it. Maybe this means looking to others for help in developing a skill so you can take an action step. Whatever it is, big or small action steps are necessary. These steps tell your heart – the whole Universe – that you are serious about something, that it means a lot to you, and that you are willing to do what needs to be done.

Your purpose exists at a soul level. Puran Bair states that we are born with a template – a seal on our soul – and that is our purpose. Your purpose is inside your heart as the heart is the gateway to the soul; you just need to access it. As you heal what covers your purpose, you get closer and closer to it. You also get closer to it by following your heart's guidance and taking action steps. So, what exactly are your action steps? Keep working on this and taking some sort of action every day. Don't forget to reward yourself in ways that nurture the present you as well as the younger you. Love yourself and celebrate all of your accomplishments, big and small.

Please keep doing the automatic writing until you are satisfied. It may take more than once if you are not used to doing it. After you write, it's time to meditate. You have all the skills now to create your own meditation. Whatever guidance you receive in your automatic writing, you want to breathe it into every chakra – especially the heart chakra and throat chakra. Give yourself the time and space to breathe in everything you received into your being, and notice what happens in your chakras and in your being. Notice what feels good or positive and what doesn't. Whatever feels positive is an action step worth pursuing, and I suggest you schedule that in and do it as soon as possible. Any small thing you can do right away, just do it! Whatever doesn't feel so good or positive may require further exploration. First, check to see if it is normal fear or resistance coming up. If it is fear or resistance, you can meditate and breathe into it wherever it is located in the body or a particular chakra. If it is not fear or resistance, it may not be in your best interest, or it could be indicative of further healing before you can initiate the action. To further discern what is worth pursuing and what is not, I encourage you to do the automatic writing again on the one particular thing you are questioning and/or meditate on it. Bring the idea into all your chakras saying love and light, and when you get to the heart chakra, notice the emotions there. When you feel deeply into the emotions, if the emotions are difficult or uncomfortable, just breathe through them, and I promise you will get clarity. When you reach the throat chakra, breathe the emotions here as well, and once you get through them, exhale the idea forward and see how that feels. Keep doing it until you feel the energy of love and light accompanying the idea. And then pursue it as soon as you can.

Some of the resistance that comes up in us may come up more than once. When I started writing this book, the question arose numerous times, asking myself, "Who do you think you are to write a book?" I healed whatever it was that came up for me, and it eventually come back again not because the healing wasn't successful but because I healed it at one level and had to go deeper to heal it at another level. Eventually, the question changed to, "Who am I to *not* write this book?"

Taking action steps is a process you will hopefully be in for the rest of your life toward your purpose. You are headed in one direction, toward one thing. This is one purpose that may include multiple facets. While you may only have a feeling around it or a clear picture, it doesn't matter as much as the fact that you can begin to take steps.

Using your neck pain level as an obvious indicator to where you are at with your purpose is most helpful. If you don't feel neck pain, you are likely on track. Look closely. If neck pain or discomfort surfaces again, it usually means you have made progress and there is healing required at a deeper level.

The previous "living from your deathbed" meditation is another helpful method to understand what the giant steps toward your purpose are. You can try to imagine yourself on your deathbed, knowing well what you wish you did or did not do in your life. The action steps you know you could have taken become clear. Hindsight is best sight, so use your hindsight to give yourself the guidance today and then take those steps, meditating through anything and everything that holds you back.

Giant Steps Chakra Meditation

Sitting in your posture with your spine ever so straight, lifting your crown up toward the ceiling, take on the Full Rhythmic Breath. Call in your spiritual support and feel their presence. Set your intention for this meditation and what you would like to get out of it regarding taking giant steps toward purpose. Using the mantra, love and light, breathe into your heart chakra, located along the inside of the spine at the back of your chest and then as you exhale, let the love and light expand your heart chakra. Continue expanding your heart chakra with each breath until it feels like you are sitting inside your heart chakra, filled with all the love and light of the whole Universe.

This will take a number of repetitions so give yourself the gift of time.

Feel yourself as your heart center and just how radiant you are.

Starting with the root chakra, breathe love and light into the chakra, allowing it to expand on the exhale. Focusing all your attention there, bring your awareness to all the changes that have transpired in the root chakra through your meditations. Breathe into all the healing, all the symbolism, characteristics, emotions, memories, sensations and meaning of the root chakra. Feel into how this chakra has evolved since you began this short but intense journey. As you continue to expand the root chakra with the breath, ask what the most important giant step forward is, that you can take right now and would contribute to your throat chakra shining brightly. It is definitely in there and may present as an image, words, sensation, emotion, or combination of experiences. Once you get clarity on a giant step toward purpose, imagine yourself doing it, getting through it to completion. Let yourself feel the process and feel your success! Write it down before you go onto the sacral chakra.

Repeat this for each of the chakras, getting in touch with all the change that has occurred in each chakra and then opening to what is next, the best giant step toward purpose. Trust in this process as much as you are able. If what comes feels great, follow through, taking that action step, completing it as soon as possible. If what comes feels awkward, try to trust and do it anyway or meditate further in that chakra until you receive further clarity or do more healing if that is needed.

Take your time with each chakra in this meditation or meditate on one chakra every day this week. Repeat this practice as many times as you want.

Working with the chakras in this way and then taking the giant steps to move forward will automatically help you feel much more alive with a new enthusiastic attitude toward life and why you are here. Your purpose will become clearer and clearer as time goes on. Your throat chakra cannot help but shine in a whole new way.

You definitely want to keep taking steps. It is one thing to gain understanding, to heal and get clarity or guidance around how to move forward, and another thing to follow through. We don't want to be all talk or all feeling! We want to move forward with giant steps toward purpose. How do we do that? Whatever we come up with in our meditations regarding small or big steps we need to take, the next most important thing is to take those steps. When I received the guidance to write this book, it would have been very easy and even normal to let the idea slide away. Not now, I will do it later. There is no later! It's important to take action because taking action keeps the energy of the discoveries in meditation flowing. Do something right away, and what you can't do in that moment, put it in your calendar, making it a priority. The energy we feel around a discovery or guidance in a meditation is so powerful, and by acting immediately, we can bring it into manifestation. We need to manifest who we are and not just think about it. If you are having trouble taking your steps, get the help or support you need. I am happy to work with you and love to help people keep taking steps forward.

Please remember that light shines on the darkness. You have been shining the light on your darkness and all that you need to change within yourself, so you can move forward and become the beautiful, shining light that you are. The neck issues that you experienced were the darkness and the healing you did in the light. Your giant steps forward are a continuation of the light as well as a manifestation of your throat chakra shining. As you continue to take giant steps forward, a new bit of darkness may surface. When this happens, you can access your tool kit of practices to bring that into the light as well. How bright can you make your throat chakra shine in this lifetime? Every time we take a giant step forward, we find ourselves in a new place of being, we are different in some way, and this is always worth celebrating. If you keep moving forward, then there will likely be a new challenge. You may wonder, does it ever end? I don't know that it does, but I will say that it gets easier and easier over time. In the beginning, it seems it is hard, and we experience so many challenges, so much darkness in between the moments of light. Eventually, it becomes the reverse, and we experience a lot more light, love, and joy, and the darkness shows itself occasionally and is much easier to move through.

I suggest that every time you take an intentional step forward that you pay attention to how it feels, celebrate the success, and feel your joy. Then, take the time to meditate on the step once you have taken it. This allows you to completely process and integrate it. Breathe the light and love into your chakras, and see what you notice, going with whatever shows up. Continuing to meditate in this way, especially focused on the giant step you just completed, will often provide for you the next natural step. Eventually, your spiritual journey and taking giant steps forward becomes very natural.

We have explored different ways to get closer and closer to your unique purpose and how to awaken to your true self. We have learned to open to more guidance by using automatic writing. You understand resistance may come up, and you now have a great toolbox full of tools to work through it so that you need not continue to suffer with neck issues. You understand the value of taking giant steps forward and how they make your throat chakra shine.

In the next chapter, you will become aware of the inevitable obstacles that will come up. You are human and if everything were straight forward and easy, you wouldn't grow. You grow through overcoming obstacles.

Chapter 15:

What Is Holding You Back?

*"Obstacles don't have to stop you. If you run into
a wall, don't turn around and give up. Figure out
how to climb it, go through it, or work around it."*
—Michael Jordan

Congratulations on making it this far into this book. Congratulations on doing some self-exploration, whether you did the practices or not. I am so curious to know where you are at now with your neck pain and throat chakra, and to know what's been holding you back in life and what, if any, steps you are taking forward in your self-expression and/ or toward your purpose. How close are you to becoming your true self, and how is your desire to become all that you truly are?

We all learn to say no as toddlers; it gives the toddler a sense of personal power. "No" is said to them, and they feel the power of the other in saying it, so they try it on for themselves. Hopefully, through life, we learn that saying "no" to life disempowers us and saying "yes" to life empowers us. I invite you to say "yes" to everything and, while doing so, discover where your "nos" are. Years ago from a friend who was trying to say "yes" to everything – all the good, the bad, and the in-between – I learned that when we say "yes," we say yes to God. On the other hand, when we say "no," we say "no" to God. While it's often easy to say "yes" to the easy things, we often later find them challenging, and then we say "no." Saying "yes" to someone yelling at you doesn't mean you have to take the yelling. Instead, you can say "yes" to the fact that they are yelling and you feel offended, and you can say "yes" to honoring yourself and removing yourself from the situation. Saying "no" reduces the flow and the opportunities, and by not acting on the difficulties and challenges in ways that serve our growth, we remain where we are.

I don't totally buy into my friend's philosophy of saying "yes" to everything one hundred percent of the time, as sometimes my choice is "No, that doesn't work for me," and I move onto something that does, but I think the general idea of it is helpful. I do like change. Do you like change? Most people like to keep everything the same, as the status quo becomes comfortable and that feeds into that built-in sense of survival. When we take risks, feel the fear, and do it anyway, we reprogram our system to see that we will survive change. We will still be here tomorrow if we do something different today. I used to be one of those people who liked things to stay the same even though I didn't realize it. I stayed in my first marriage way too long for this reason. It was when I left the marriage and started making changes in my life that

I saw things improve, and while I didn't always make the best choices and nothing was ever prefect, I learned to take risks. There is so much written today from successful people who had to fail multiple times before they succeeded. You know it is all about the journey, not the goal.

To me, success is about overcoming all the obstacles within myself, clearing all that gets in the way within myself – whatever is inside me preventing me from living my dreams and becoming who I truly am. I learned that my own resistance, in whatever form it comes in, is there to serve me, so I say "yes" to my resistance. I've been around this block thousands of times, and it serves me so well. By feeling into my resistance, I move beyond it.

Years ago, I first started getting strong guidance in my meditations, I would often say "no" to it, thinking, "That can't be real; I couldn't possibly do that," and so on. I would usually come around and see the truth in it much later, but I also saw how I wasted a great deal of time. I learned that I resisted whatever was good for me; what an epiphany that was. So, I changed my approach. I decided that whenever I got guidance to do something or pursue something and I resisted it, I would do it anyway. I started to do whatever I resisted. I don't know about you, but resistance to my own growth has been huge, and while I still experience resistance to this day, I deal with it much differently than I did in my younger days. Resistance is normal; it's what we do with it that matters.

Are you feeling any resistance to using this book, the practices, and the message in it to heal your neck pain and move forward in your life? Maybe you're not sure if you have resistance or not. Some of the resistance you might be experiencing could look like this:

- You like to meditate but don't have the time to do it every day.

- You don't have enough experience with these practices.

- You're not as spiritual as you thought you were.

- Your problem is too big.

- You've tried everything, and this will likely be just another thing that fails.

- This is just way too much for you.

- You're afraid you won't be able to do it.

- Your physical pain stops you from meditating for long.

- You're not disciplined enough.

- You need my help but can't afford it financially.

- If you change too much, what will your partner, friends, or family think?

- Some of this stuff is way too out there for me.

Does any of this sound familiar? Trust me, I felt every one of these and more, and if I can move beyond them, so can you. Maybe it's true that this book and its message is not for you. Maybe you just need to move on to something else and pass this along, and that is totally fine. I appreciate it greatly that you stayed with me to this point.

I watched an old interview on YouTube with Pir Vilayat. He was a great Sufi master, son of Hazrat Inayat Khan, and near the end of the video, he asked the question, "What if?" If you ponder anything here and wonder if it's possible that maybe some of this will work for you or, better still, that you have tried some of the practices and you like them, I invite you to ask yourself, "What if?"

I invite you to make your own list of resistant thoughts or feelings. Write them all down or type them on your computer. Better still, use the automatic writing method and see what all comes out. Don't be surprised if it is a long list. If it's a short list, feel me bowing at your feet!

Write your list, as I did above, and come back to it the next day and see if there is anything you need to add or take away. I encourage you to reword each item on your list by starting it with "What if?" Here is the list I provided reworded:

- What if I like to meditate and I can create the time to do it every day?

- What if I actually do have enough experience to keep going?

- What if I am even more spiritual than I think I am?

- What if my problem is not too big after all?

- What if I've tried everything and this just might be the one thing that works?

- What if this is not way too much for me?

- What if *I can* do it?

- What if I find ways to help my comfort level when meditating?

- What if I find ways to be disciplined enough?

- What if you want my personal help and discover you actually can afford it?

- What if you change a lot and your partner, friends, or family think you're even more amazing?

- What if some of this stuff is actually a perfect vehicle for you to change?

How do you feel at the end of reading the first list, and how do you feel at the end of reading the second list? While we face the unknown, we can still step into it. I can't tell you how many times I made big changes in my life, and I went through a time of feeling lost in the dark. I can't promise you that if you follow my program you won't ever feel lost in the dark, that it won't be hard, that you won't get frustrated, or that all kind of uncomfortable things will likely come up. I won't even say I wish I could make it easy for you because I wouldn't be honoring your soul if I did. Your soul knew what it was getting into, and your soul knows that all the challenges you face in this life are there to help you grow to become who you truly are and fulfill your purpose. Your neck pain is one of these challenges. As it did in my experience, neck pain has to get that bad before you say, "Okay, enough already; let me look at this from another perspective and see what else I can do." I invite you to honor your soul and your soul's purpose, even if you aren't aware of what all that means. Honor the fact that your soul is an extension of God, just like the sun's rays are an extension of the sun.

I invite you to work this book, flag your favorite pages, highlight and underline, and make it yours. Go back and read the whole thing and put your all into it. You are worth it; you deserve to be the change you want to see. Feel the people who want your help pulling at you. Tune into their hearts and their longing for your help. You answered my call to let me help you. You can work this book to the max, or you can work with me directly. I accept whatever choice you make, but please work through your resistance before you make your choice. If you don't work through your resistance, the same issues will come up for any kind of help. Once you work through it, I know you will make the best decision for yourself. I have been an independent woman most of my life and I used to pride myself on that thinking I was pretty strong. Sure, I am strong, but for me, it actually takes more courage to ask for help then receive it. It takes more courage to work with others, and the strength I gained in living my life from a place of openness and connection to others is immeasurable.

In the past, I didn't think that I was meant to help others, that I was meant to make a real difference, or that healing myself and growing was all I could handle, and even more than I could handle. I realize now that as I healed and grew, the people around me healed and grew. So, even if you don't know whether or not you are meant to help others, what if you are meant to help yourself? Whether your self needs you, others need you, or the world needs you, I encourage you to discover whether or not it's right for you to open up and go deeper into this work. I promise that if you do, you will change. You will not stay the same, and your life will begin to change. I can also promise you that if all your neck pain doesn't go away, you will at the least experience some long-term relief from it. I can promise you that your relationships will improve, and I can promise you that you will begin to experience more joy and satisfaction. I invite you to move beyond your pain and throat chakra issues and move forward in the life you are destined to live.

I was born to help you. It's no coincidence that I have the following qualifications, as at some level – maybe even as deep as the soul level – you knew my skills would serve you:

+ Meditating for twenty-five years and teaching meditation for fifteen years

+ Practiced shamanism and then Heart-Centered Shamanism for over twenty years

+ Certification in Hurqalya Healing, Jin Shin Do Acupressure, Reiki Master, HRM Retreat, Guide and HRM Teacher, Mentor, and Coach

+ Developed Heart-Centered Shamanism

+ Studied many spiritual and healing modalities

+ Brought all my past training and experience together to help you heal your neck pain and throat chakra issues so you can move forward in your life

Let's do a quick little meditation to see if this book or my program is meant for you.

I invite you to get into the meditative posture and take on the full, rhythmic breath. Call in your spiritual support. Breathe all the light and love of the whole Universe into your heart chakra. Proceed to do the same with all your chakras, and when it feels right ask yourself if this book or my program is meant for you. If it is not, I thank you from deep in my heart for reading to the end. If my book or my program are meant for you, ask your heart if it is ideal for you to work through the book on your own or work with me directly to eliminate your neck pain and move forward in your life at a much faster pace and let your throat chakra shine.

Thank you for being brave enough to look at what may be holding you back in your journey to healing your neck issues and letting your throat chakra shine. By looking at what might be getting in the way, you move into a form of empowerment. By facing the obstacles on your path and acknowledging they are there, you can say yes to yourself. I know what's ahead and that allows us to make that commitment or deepen an existing commitment to the self in spite of one's obstacles.

Chapter 16:

Now Is the Time

"Let your light shine so brightly that others can
see their way out of the dark."

—Katrina Mayer

My wish at this point is that you healed your neck pain or at the very least reduced it significantly. In addition to healing your neck pain, my wish is that you moved forward in your life in ways you dreamed of or, better still, beyond what you dreamed. You deserve to live pain-free and live your purpose with joy and happiness. My wish is that this book and these practices opened doors of self-discovery and you know yourself more intimately and gained a new sense of self compassion and self-love. I hope that this book helped you experience healing in many different ways along with the self-empowerment you were born to experience. I hope that you accessed the light and love that you are and are now shining in ways you weren't aware existed.

You immersed yourself in something quite intense and my deepest wish is that you reaped benefits beyond your expectations. You have been able to commit to yourself and this program, strengthening yourself in ways that you want to continue. You created a sense of safety that enables fears of the past to fall away. This sense of safety may branch out into other areas of your life and you feel a confidence to take risks that was hidden in the shadows previously.

You had the courage and fortitude to learn new meditation practices with energy healing and Heart-Centered Shamanism. Your existing knowledge of the chakras has expanded to include your own personal experiences of the chakras, their location, how they feel, what colors or shapes are associated with them, and how to work beautifully with love and light in these centers. You developed the skills to uncover your own past hurts that held you back, along with the skills to heal anything and everything that came up for you physically, emotionally, and energetically. My hope is that you will continue to use these practices and possibly even learn more or even develop your own for your continued healing and empowerment.

You worked hard on all your chakras, creating the foundation for change and then hitting the ball out of the park with your throat chakra, appreciating the importance of this work to create the change you wanted to see and be. Through all of it, you kept going, not giving up, and through this intense chakra work, you deepened your relationship with self with greater understanding, compassion, and love. You healed your inner child and likely even changed the past, which made you into more of the person you truly are.

You opened yourself to Heart-Centered Shamanism, and through practices with Power Animals and/or spirits in nature, you developed a growing connection with the entire Universe and all that it contains. We are not separate; we are all One, and this understanding is beginning to take up residence in your being.

You learned to access much within yourself that was hidden and now you are free to let your light shine in its own unique ways. You can hold your head high knowing that you began a process working toward your soul's purpose. There is a level of trust in you that was hard to feel before. This level of trust changes everything, and you can now celebrate the unfolding of the real you.

By doing the practices in this book and integrating the teachings, you came so far. I appreciate all your efforts and know how difficult it is. You are worth it, and your process is so worthwhile.

I don't want to see you playing small anymore. I did that for *way* too long. Even when I realized how small I played, it took me a decade to totally step out of that behavior, and a decade is not necessary. I wrote this book so you don't have to suffer anymore. Your neck pain is but a symptom of a much deeper problem; your neck pain manifested when you were ready to look inward. Your pain is an expression of something inside you that wants to heal and is ready to heal.

My wish for you goes beyond healing your neck pain and moving forward in your life. My wish for you is that you *become all that you can be*. I want you to fully and completely access all your *light*, *extract* the magnificent and *divine you* so that *you* can *shine*. This is my deepest wish for you. Please read this over and over and close your eyes while breathing my words into your heart.

If this book helped you in ways you hoped for, please continue to do the practices so that the world can benefit more and more for having you in it.

Know I am here to help you in any way I can.

Thank You

Thank you, thank you, for opening yourself to reading this book, for having the courage to do the meditations and staying the path. I am deeply grateful you made it to the end of this book, and my wish for you is that you learned much about yourself and have benefited in ways you were not expecting.

I will hold you in my heart with the vision that you become all that you truly are and that your throat chakra shines beyond your wildest dreams!

If you have questions for me, please contact me at cheryl-stelte.com or through my Facebook group – Shining Throat Chakras, Healing and Empowerment to Soul Purpose

About the Author

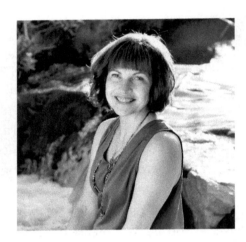

Cheryl Stelte is a spiritual teacher, healer, coach, and author who helps people transform themselves and their lives, accessing and expressing the truth of who they truly are and why they are here. After twenty-five years of spiritual practice, study, and teaching, Cheryl is grateful to dedicate herself to helping others access their soul's purpose and shine their light in the world.

Cheryl was drawn to meditation early on, and over the last twenty-five years has studied, practiced, and taught various forms of meditation. Her initial motivator was to heal her own severe depression; she soon got off anti-depressants and never went back.

Her spiritual journey and her love of the forests, mountains, and oceans drew Cheryl to shamanism, where she trained through the Foundation for Shamanic Studies and with other shamanic teachers. She has since developed Heart-Centered Shamanism.

Cheryl is certified through IAMHeart as a teacher, mentor, coach, personal retreat guide, and Hurqalya Energy Healing practitioner. She holds diplomas in acupressure (Cdn. Acupressure College), fashion design (Blanche MacDonald); certificates in interior design (Victoria, BC), elemental space clearing (Denise Linn), hatha yoga teaching; and is a reiki master (India). She achieves great success in helping others heal and become empowered.

Cheryl is a Canadian living in Denver, Colorado with her husband Amin. She has two wonderful grown children, Dan and Charla, and enjoys hiking, kayaking, French cooking and decor, and most of all, helping others shine their light.

ABOUT THE AUTHOR

CPSIA information can be obtained
at www.ICGtesting.com
Printed in the USA
JSHW021255110221
11794JS00004B/207